CORE EXERCISES
FOR SENIORS

Build Strength and Improve Stability for Active Aging After 60

Baz Thompson

TABLE OF CONTENTS

BEFORE YOU START READING

As a special gift, I included a logbook and my book, "Strength Training After 40" (regularly priced at $16.97 on Amazon) and the best part is, you get access to all of them.

FREE

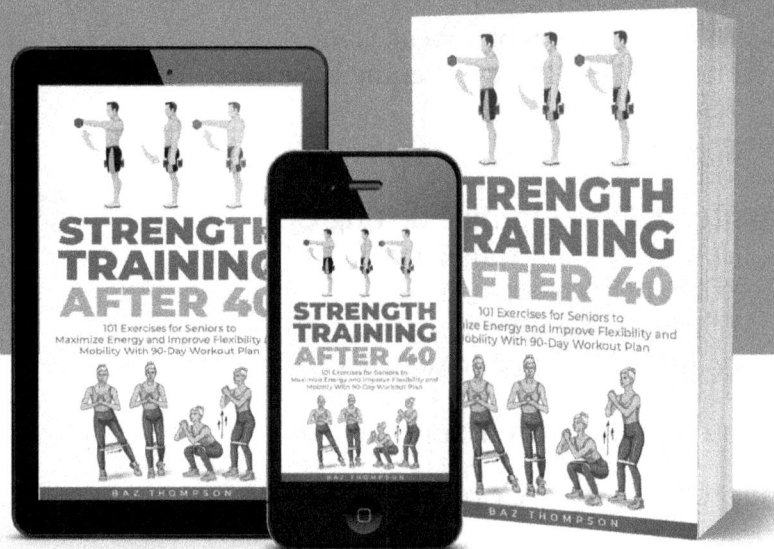

WHAT'S IN IT FOR ME?

- 101 highly effective strength training exercises that can help you reach the highest point of your fitness performance
- Foundational exercises to improve posture and increase range of motion in your arms, shoulders, chest, and back
- Stretches to help you gain flexibility and find deep relaxation
- Workout Logbook to help you keep track of your accomplishments and progress. Log your progress to give you the edge you need to accomplish your goals.

SCAN ME

INTRODUCTION

You are looking forward to growing older with vitality and grace. But maybe you aren't sure how to achieve that. The good news is that you are reading this book. That means that you are hungry for information and willing to learn! In this instructional and practical guide, you will learn all about one of the pillars of active aging: a strong core.

Along with balance, strength, and flexibility, core strength is something you don't want to grow older lacking. You may currently have a weak or compromised abdominal and back muscle because of injury or surgery. On the other hand, perhaps you have a moderately strong core and want to take preventative measures to keep that strength as you age. Regardless of where you are physically, you can benefit from strengthening your core through exercise. We will travel this road together, learning about our bodies, how to keep them strong, and what simple choices we can make to ensure that we age well.

What are some everyday tasks that our core helps us to achieve? Just about everything!

- Sitting in a chair
- Getting up from the floor, bed, or chair
- Turning to look behind you
- Picking up items, bags, or packages
- Bending over to tie your shoes
- Getting dressed
- Taking a bath or shower
- Reaching for items overhead
- Vacuuming, mopping, sweeping
- Hammering, cutting, turning a screwdriver
- Physical activities like swimming, biking, bowling, golfing, tennis, rowing, running, walking

Our core must remain strong to retain our capacity to do these basic tasks. If not, we may require the assistance of others and lose our ability to live and work independently.

All our muscles, including those in our core, gradually lose mass and strength as we get older. While some of this may be due to injuries, surgeries, or illnesses, we often lose muscle strength because of inactivity. As a result, we fail or forget to train and work the muscles we need to stay strong. The good news? With regular exercise, we can regain and maintain strength in our muscles, particularly our core muscles.

ABOUT THIS BOOK

We will cover a lot of ground in this book, but it is all practical and easy-t0-understand information. The first part of the book helps develop a foundational understanding of our bodies, particularly our core. The second part of the book comprises the actual core exercises, broken down by the position in which they are done. And the last part of the book includes the practical application.

- In Chapter 1, we will see a brief overview of aging and how we can slow the loss of muscle mass. Also covered is an outline of the core muscles and how a strong core benefits our daily living. Finally, there is a quick core strength quiz to help you assess your condition.

- Chapter 2 goes into how we can develop core strength. No special equipment is needed! Common mistakes are revealed and helpful tips for making the most of your exercise time.

- Mat core exercises are the focus in Chapter 3. Do you think this chapter is all about sit-ups? Think again! Featured are twelve of the best core exercises you can do while lying down.

Spoiler alert: no sit-ups or crunches are involved.

- In Chapter 4, seated core exercises are the focus. Many people are surprised to learn how safe, low-impact, and effective seated exercises can be for people of any age. Twelve powerful core exercises are highlighted and can all be done in a chair.

- Chapter 5 concentrates on standing core exercises and training your core muscles while standing gives you the element of surprise. It mixes up your training routine and allows muscles to be worked differently. Spotlighted are twelve standing core strengtheners.

- If you have a spouse, partner, or workout buddy, you will enjoy Chapter 6. This section is devoted to core exercises that you can do with a partner. These eight exercises are challenging and fun.

- Chapter 7 calls attention to warm-up exercises and cool down stretches. These can be easy to overlook or forget, but it's essential to take a few minutes before exercising to prime our bodies and after exercising to let them unwind.

- Chapter 8 outlines one of the primary ways to exercise and work our core: walking! There is a brief description of the best walking tips, along with six of the best ways to incorporate core exercises into your daily walk.

- The action plan is revealed in Chapter 9. There are three weeks of workout routines for you to choose from or work through in this chapter.

Each week features six days of core exercises.

HOW TO USE THIS BOOK

Not only will you learn about your core and the benefits of a strong core, but you will also find fifty core exercises that you can start doing today. In addition, there are ten exercises to help you get warmed up and cooled down. This book can be used as a guidebook and reference that you can turn back to again and again as you learn to strengthen your core.

Each exercise in this book will feature the following:

- Name of the exercise
- Time needed per rep
- Total time to complete the exercise
- Easy step-by-step instructions
- A variation of the exercise or a way to level up and make the exercise more challenging
- Safety tips and things to watch out for to avoid injury

Illustrations accompanying each exercise will show you the correct positioning of your body, head, hands, and feet.

You can use this book in various ways, depending on your interests, abilities, and needs. One way is to work through each exercise, one-by-one, chapter-by-chapter systematically. Another way is to make up your exercise routine, picking the exercises you want to do each day. Or, to make life easy, you can take advantage of the weekly schedules at the end of the book and follow these. Find a system that you can stick to and that works for you. A stronger core awaits you and can be achieved with a bit of effort!

Getting older is unavoidable. But losing muscle mass and strength in our bodies does not have to go along with that. Becoming educated about how our bodies function, learning how we can slow down muscle loss, deciding to take steps to better our health, and putting in the effort to follow through with action will determine whether we age well or age. In writing this book, one of my goals is to encourage you on your health and well-being journey. So, we can all enjoy an active and strong second half of our lives. I hope that you will find this book a helpful resource as you strengthen your core and build your stability.

Please consult with your doctor before starting on any new exercise or activity.

Please accept my heartfelt gratitude for downloading my book. Please leave a review on Amazon to let me know what you think. This will benefit a lot of other individuals who are looking for a book like mine. To me, that would be really valuable.

Scan the QR Code To Leave a Review:

My hope and desire is that you will find this book to be a valuable resource as you struggle to regain and maintain good balance in order to avoid falls and improve your general health. Are you all set? Let's get your fitness education and training started!

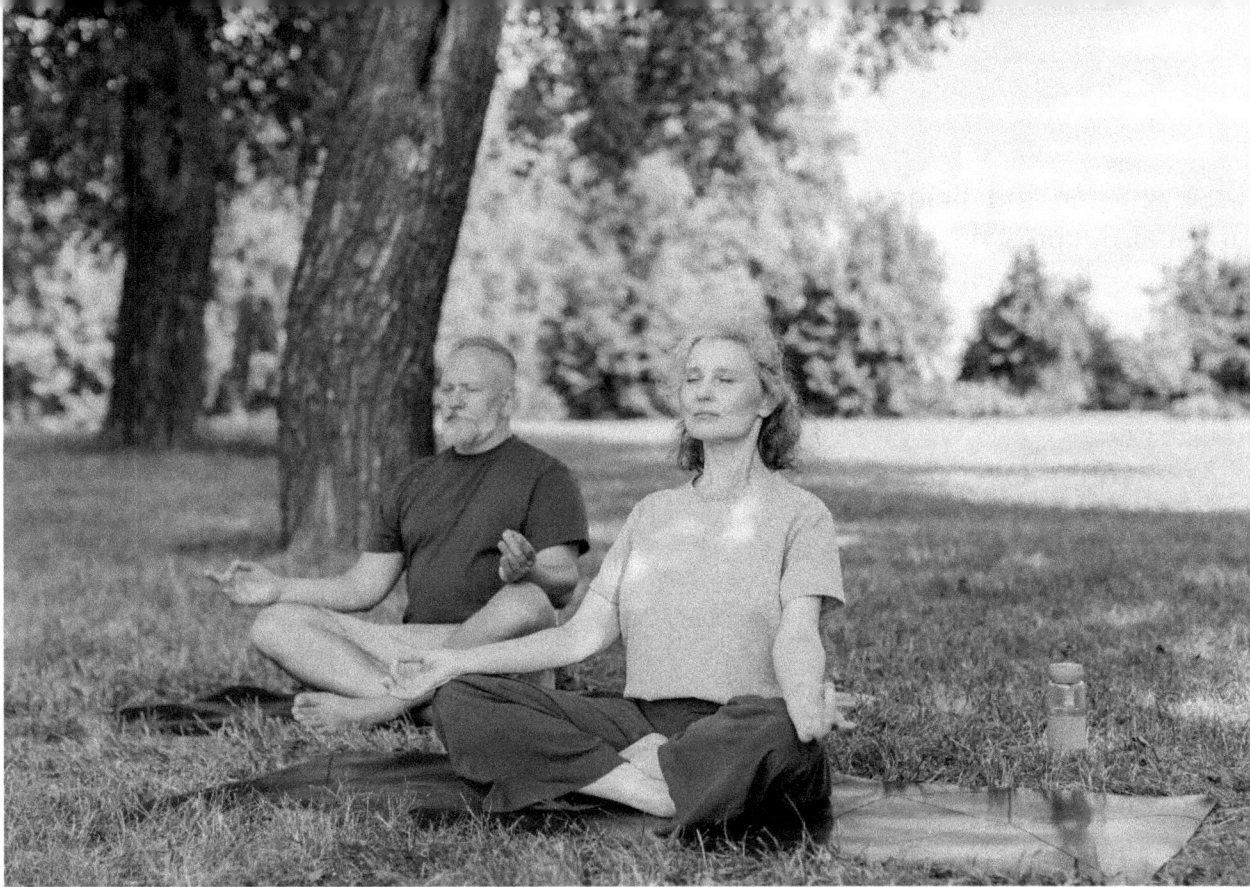

Age is inevitable. Aging isn't. —Marv Levy

Chapter 1:
The Power of Your Core

Strong core muscles are a crucial part of our health and well-being. But they are also important to keep us physically mobile and stable. Our stability ensures that we can do certain tasks without the assistance of others as we get older. This helps us to stay independent for a longer period of time. In this chapter, we will take a brief look at what happens to our bodies as we progress in years. Next, we will examine what muscles make up our core muscles. We will define the benefits of having a strong core. Finally, there is a short quiz that can help determine whether our core is strong or lacking.

OUR BODIES AND AGING

Getting older is a natural part of life. However, once we hit 60 years of age, we may be labeled as old. This was perhaps true in the past centuries when life spans were shorter and living to age 60 was unusual. But presently, older adults live full and active lives well into their eighth and ninth decades of life. The older population is divided into three subcategories:

Young-Old (ages 65 to 74)

Middle-Old (ages 75 to 84)

Old-Old (ages 85 and older)

The physical abilities and strengths of someone who is 65 years old can vary greatly from someone who is 85 years old, depending on their mental acuity, fitness level, and overall health. Besides age, a variety of factors can contribute to this difference, including foods eaten, exercise, weight, enriching activities, and adequate sleep.

Chronological age is something we cannot control, but biological age is reflected by the choices we make. For example, a 72-year-old may have battled breast cancer. This person chooses to consume a diet consisting of lean proteins, fresh fruits, and fresh vegetables. They can still play golf twice a week, practice stretching exercises daily, and complete jigsaw puzzles regularly. Another 72-year-old may suffer from a little arthritis in the hands and not have any other major health issues but chooses to eat a diet high in processed foods, salt, and sugar. They have constant brain fog, don't exercise, and spend most of their day sitting inside watching television. These two 72-year-olds are the same age chronologically, but biologically they are aging at different rates.

The human body is composed of many different types of cells. Some are short-lived and constantly being replaced, like skin cells. Others are long-lived but are never replaced, like brain cells. Muscle cells are self-renewing. As we age, however, we lose muscle mass and strength, contributing to increased frailty and instability. Slowing down the loss of muscle can be achieved with just a few changes in our lifestyle. A 2018 study by McCormick and Vasilaki recommended paying attention to the following factors to help maintain muscle mass and strength:

- Increased protein intake. Nearly 40% of people over 50 years old do not consume adequate amounts of protein.

- Aerobic exercise. Walking, running, cycling, and swimming stimulate the heart and blood flow to muscles while increasing lung capacity.

- Resistance training. Lifting weights, bodyweight exercise, and resistance bands stimulate skeletal muscles to grow and become stronger.

- Other physical activities. Stretching, yoga, and core exercises bring flexibility and strength to muscles.

Choosing to make changes to our daily life can help slow the loss of muscle strength and core stability as we grow older.

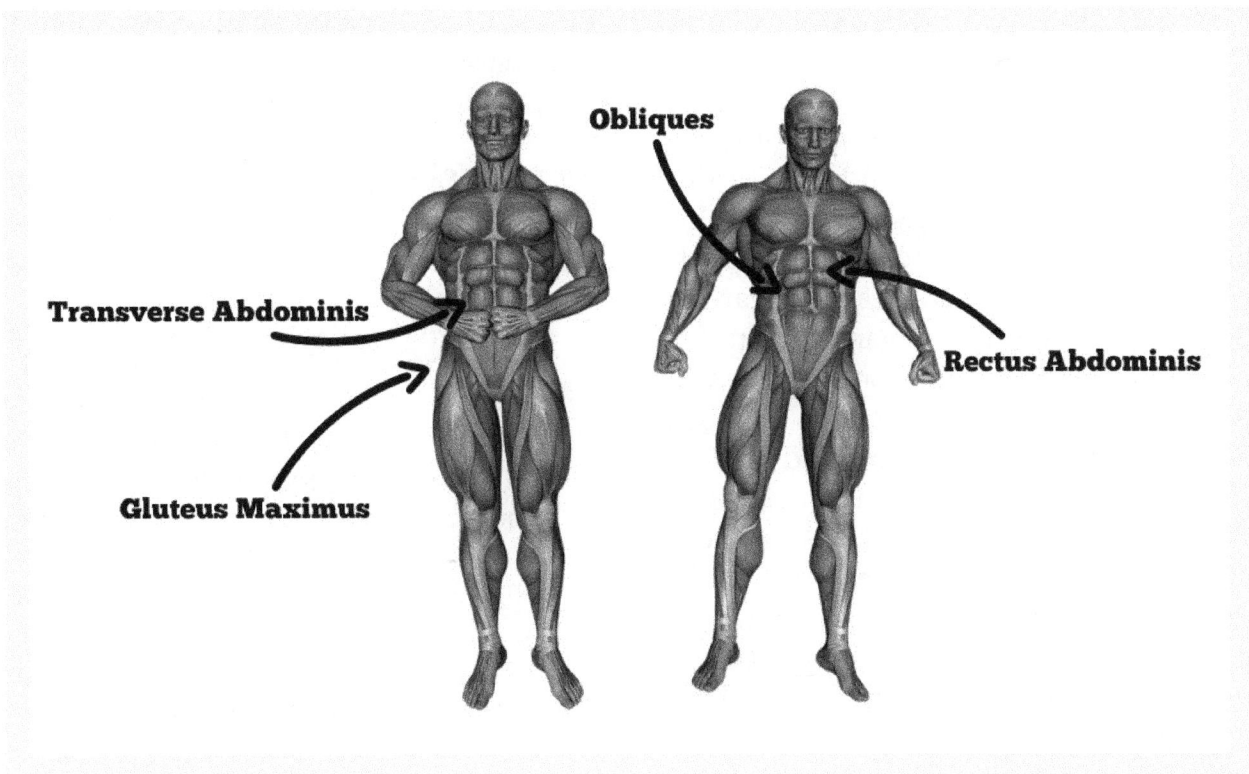

Obliques

Transverse Abdominis

Gluteus Maximus

Rectus Abdominis

WHAT IS YOUR CORE

It is common to think that your core is just your abdominal muscles. Your abs are definitely part of your core, but there are nearly 35 muscles that make up this "torso girdle" that supports the body.

The main core muscles include:

- Rectus abdominis. This is what most people think of as "6 pack muscles" at the front of your abdomen. These muscles run from under your rib cage to your pubic bone.

- Obliques. Internal and external oblique muscles are on the sides of your torso. These muscles help you twist and turn your body.

- Transverse abdominis. This muscle holds your pelvis and internal organs in place.

- Erector spinae. These muscles are in your back along the spine and help you stand erect.

- Gluteus maximus. Located in your buttocks, these muscles assist you in lifting your legs, walking, and climbing stairs.

This brief overview gives you an idea of what some of these muscles do in supporting the body. There are several other core muscles not mentioned here that also play an important role.

THE RISK FACTORS OF A WEAK CORE

Lisa was a mother and grandmother that enjoyed being around her family. One of her favorite things to do with her granddaughters was to teach them how to plant flowers and vegetables in the garden. She had learned how to garden from her grandmother and loved working the earth to yield beautiful blooms and produce. At one time, Lisa was an avid dancer, but because of occasional arthritis in her knees, she did not dance as much anymore. In fact, she shied away from exercise of any kind because she did not enjoy the repetitive movements of most exercise routines. She preferred the freer expression of dance. One weekend, Lisa was lifting a heavy bag of potting soil from the trunk of her car and lost her balance. She fell in her driveway. Her arm braced her as she fell, but it was broken in two places as a result of landing on the concrete. Lisa spent the next few months recuperating from a broken arm, unable to garden with her granddaughters.

In the United States, one out of four older adults falls annually. Twenty-six million falls were reported in 2018, and that number increases from year to year. Falls are the leading cause of injury in adults over the age of 65 and are blamed for millions of injuries. What is causing older adults to fall? There are a variety of reasons, including impaired eyesight, slower reflexes, medications that cause dizziness, tripping hazards, and low blood pressure. Another primary reason for falls is the loss of balance and stability resulting from a weak core. The strength and flexibility of our back, abdominal, and buttock muscles determine our ability to react and adjust to changes in certain situations.

Some risks of having a core that cannot support you adequately include:

1. **INCREASED PAIN:** Weak core muscles cause your pelvis to tilt and other muscles to pull on your spine, resulting in lower back and neck pain.

2. **POOR POSTURE:** Shoulders that hunch forward, a neck that cranes out, and a spine that is not in alignment are all indicators of a weak core.

3. **IMBALANCE AND INSTABILITY:** Loss of balance results from your muscles being unable to keep you supported and stable as you twist, turn, reach, and lift. These imbalances can lead to falls.

4. **FATIGUE:** Loss of breath, inability to lift or carry items and overall sense of weakness are indicators of weak core muscles.

Loss of strength and stamina in your core muscles can infringe on your abilities and overall well-being.

THE BENEFITS OF STRENGTHENING YOUR CORE

Debbie and Tom loved camping. They both enjoyed the outdoors and had gone camping since they first started dating in the 1970s. As they raised their children, they did plenty of tent camping and taught their kids how to set up tents, haul water, and make a campfire. Once Tom turned 65, they decided to splurge and buy an RV so they could travel and camp all along the coastline. Debbie and Tom were both active in their local paddleball club and played several times a week.

Even though they were in their early 70s, they didn't have any trouble driving their RV, maneuvering up and down the vehicle stairs, or reaching up to secure the awnings when they packed up, thanks to their legs and core muscles being strong.

It is easy to take our core muscles for granted. But someone with impaired abdominal and back muscles would have had a difficult time doing some of the things in the above scenario. Going up and down narrow stairs, lifting and lowering awnings, and even handling a larger recreational vehicle can be tiring and possibly hazardous for someone who lacks core strength.

Is having a strong core the same as having well-defined six-pack abs? Not exactly. Having a strong core is more than just a nice physical appearance. Training and building your core muscles results in real-life benefits that affect your overall quality of life. Let's look at some of the benefits of having a well-toned core.

1. **REDUCED PAIN:** Other areas of your body, such as the lower back and neck, don't have to compensate when the muscles that support your midsection and back are toned and strong.
2. **GOOD POSTURE:** The muscles in your back and on the sides of your body, as well as the inner core muscles that attach to your spine, help you stay erect and upright.
3. **BETTER BALANCE AND STABILITY:** Having torso muscles that are sturdy helps provide a solid foundation for keeping you stable and staying on balance.
4. **INNER ORGAN PROTECTION:** The organs inside our midsection, like the stomach, liver, and kidneys, are protected by the muscles of our core. Having a muscular shield to deflect any potential damage helps keep them safe from injury.

A strong core is good for our physical bodies, but it's also central to things going smoothly in our everyday lives. Many tasks and functions are more difficult when our core muscles are not as strong as they could be. Some common everyday tasks that are helped by a strong core include:

- Driving a car
- Putting away groceries
- Exercising
- Holding a grandbaby
- Running errands
- Playing with grandkids
- Walking your dog
- Dancing with your partner

These everyday activities can be hindered or more difficult if your core muscles are not strong and flexible. A strong core contributes to maintaining a healthy and active lifestyle as you grow older. It also helps you to stay stronger longer. We all want to live independently without needing assistance.

TEST YOUR CORE

How strong is your core? You can discern if your core could benefit from strengthening by taking the quiz below. Be honest in your answers. No one is judging you or your abilities.

CORE STRENGTH QUIZ

The answer choices are: Yes or No.

1. From a seated position on the floor or a chair, can you stand up without the support of your hands or arms?

2. Does your lower back frequently hurt or feel stiff, particularly after exercise?

3. Do you often find yourself slouching, shoulders hunching forward, or noticing your posture is off?

4. Can you close your eyes and lift one foot off the floor without losing your balance?

5. Do you inadvertently hold your breath during exercises?

6. Does your midsection or lower back sag down while you are holding a plank position?

If you answered Yes to at least two questions, you would greatly benefit from training your core. These questions provide tell-tale signs that your core may be weak.

What Does the Quiz Reveal?

1. Core strength, particularly in your abdominal area, is needed to raise yourself from a lying to a seated position as well as from a seated to a standing position. If you are relying on your hands and arms to push you up, it's because your core isn't able to do that on its own.

2. Assuming that you are not suffering from a back injury, arthritis, or recovering from surgery, pain, and stiffness in your lower back may be a lack of core strength and from weak muscles around your spine.

3. Poor posture is often an indicator of insufficient core stability.

4. Balance issues can be due to a number of factors, but many times it is from a lack of core stability. Your core muscles are the ones that stabilize you as you walk, turn, and twist.

5. Holding your breath while you exercise is an indicator that your core muscles are not as strong as they could be. Your core strength is what helps you to breathe as your body works out or engages in physical activity. The inability to both breathe and move through a core exercise at the same time signals core weakness.

6. Whether it is a straight arm or modified plank, your core is what keeps your back straight during the exercise. Any sagging in your lower body is a sign that your core isn't doing its job.

Now that we know more about the core muscles, the benefits of strengthening them, and the general state of our own cores, in the next chapter, we will look at what we can do to develop a strong core.

Key Takeaways from Chapter 1:

- We can prevent the loss of muscle mass and strength that naturally occurs with aging by making a few lifestyle changes.

- The core muscles in the front, sides and back of our torso support our body and our ability to do everyday activities.

- A strong core gives us better balance and helps reduce pain.

Chapter 2:
Developing a Strong Core

We can't avoid age. However, we can avoid some aging. Continue to do things. Be active. Life is fantastic in the way it adjusts to demands; if you use your muscles and mind, they stay there much longer.

—Charles H. Townes

Remaining strong and stable is an important part of aging well. To live an active, interesting, and fulfilling life as you enter your sixties, seventies, eighties, and beyond, you must retain the ability to perform everyday tasks. Staying physically active and maintaining core strength is important if you want to continue to do the things you enjoy.

In this chapter, we will look at the fundamentals of developing a strong core. In particular, we will learn when and where to exercise plus discover what common mistakes to avoid.

HOW TO EXERCISE YOUR CORE

Training and strengthening your core is not just performing abdominal exercises. Because your core muscles run along your entire torso from under your rib cage to your pelvis, from side to side, and along your back down to your buttocks, they take up a lot of real estate on your torso. Around thirty-five muscles, both large and small, make up your core. These muscles can be worked every day, as long as you aren't working the same ones all the time. By training a variety of these muscles, you will build a solid foundation that serves as a link between the upper and lower halves of your body. This sturdy connection allows your arms and legs to do their jobs to their fullest capacity. Let's take a look at some best practices to work on your core.

WHEN TO EXERCISE

Some trainers recommend a morning routine, and others swear by exercising in the afternoon. What's the difference? Let's take a look.

Advantages of a morning exercise routine:

1. **CONSISTENT HABIT:** Getting up and lacing up your sneakers each morning builds a routine that stays consistent.

2. **BETTER SLEEP:** Working out early helps you fall asleep and stay asleep at night.

3. **LESSENS HUNGER:** You may find you are less hungry during the day if you work out in the morning.

Advantages of an afternoon exercise routine:

1. **ALREADY WARMED UP:** Unlike exercising in the morning when your body is still waking up, and muscles are stiff, an afternoon workout happens when you are fully awake and moving about.

2. **HORMONE BALANCE:** Cortisol, the stress hormone, peaks in the morning but decreases as the day goes on. On the other hand, testosterone, a muscle growth hormone, is produced at higher levels in the afternoon.

Most trainers agree that exercising at night isn't the best because it can disrupt your body's circadian rhythm or internal clock. In addition, because exercise stimulates your nervous system, you may find that working out late at night may prevent you from falling or staying asleep.

Regardless of when you choose to work out, the important thing is to try to exercise consistently at the same time every day. By making regular appointments with yourself to train and strengthen your body, you will build a habit that reaps lifetime benefits.

WHERE TO EXERCISE

There are many options to choose from when deciding where to exercise. Depending on your preference, financial situation, or comfort level, you may choose to exercise in private or public. Some options of where to perform exercises include:

• **YOUR HOME:** You may have a spare bedroom, space in your garage, or a spot in your backyard where you can comfortably exercise. The advantage of working out at home is the privacy and convenience of not having to go elsewhere. Plus, it's free. You can also work out at any time of day and aren't dependent on someone else's open hours.

- **GYM:** Whether it is a small privately-owned gym or a larger commercial gym franchise, gyms can be good places to exercise. They do have monthly fees but offer several types of cardio equipment, weight machines, free weights, and exercise classes. Many also have a trainer available to guide you through exercise routines for an additional fee. Working out at a gym can be a fun social experience and a place to connect with people.

COMMON MISTAKES TO AVOID

While core exercises aren't complicated, there are some common pitfalls to avoid. These exercises differ from those done for cardiovascular benefit, resistance training with weights, and stretching. When exercising your core, paying attention to potential mistakes when exercising your core is essential to avoid injury and discouragement.

Things to avoid when exercising your core include:

1. **POOR FORM:** Having incorrect positioning of your body, arms, or legs while performing core exercises can cause pain or injury. It also won't work the right muscles or give you the desired outcome. Poor form can sometimes be caused by the body being tired, or the exercise being too difficult.

2. **EXERCISING TOO FAST:** Rushing through core exercises to get them done quickly will not give you the results you want. Core training requires tension and time. Doing the exercises slowly and correctly is the goal.

3. **DOING TOO MUCH TOO SOON:** We all want results, and we want them right now. So, we jump in and do too much too soon! Start at a reasonable pace and add time and difficulty slowly. If you get too sore or injure yourself, you may become discouraged and quit altogether.

Key Takeaways from Chapter 2:

- Choose a consistent time to work out each day to build a regular habit.

- Find the place that you are most comfortable exercising and will stick to.

- Being aware of common pitfalls helps to avoid injury and discouragement.

We will learn the best mat, seated, and standing core exercises, in the following few chapters.

Chapter 3:
Mat Core Exercises

Don't go through life, grow through life.

— Eric Butterworth

Mat exercises are an effective way to train and strengthen your core. Most people associate mat core exercises with old-fashioned sit-ups or crunches. While sit-ups may have some merit, they aren't the best exercise for us as we get older. Sit-ups and crunches can put unnecessary strain on our spine, backs, and necks. The mat exercises outlined in this chapter concentrate on training your core while close to the floor. As you might have guessed, there is no fear of falling or losing your balance while doing these mat exercises, so they are perfect for those who may suffer from instability issues or have trouble standing or sitting. These exercises make it convenient for you to work out your core from an all-fours or reclined position. You will need a padded mat or carpeted floor to perform these.

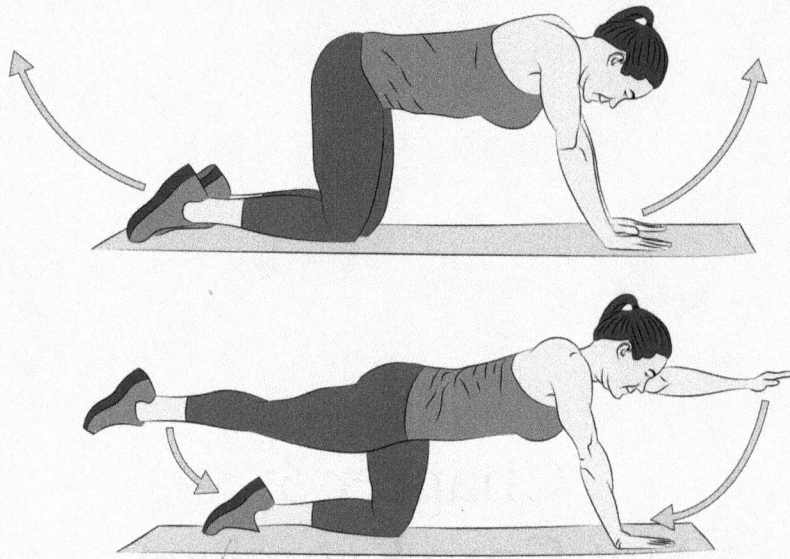

BIRD DOG

HOW TO:

1. Place hands and knees on the floor, ensuring that your hands are directly below your shoulders and knees directly below your hips.

2. Raise your right knee off the floor and extend your right foot back and up off the floor until it is parallel to the floor, if possible.

3. Now, raise your left hand off the floor and extend it out in front of you. Protect your neck by continuing to look at the floor. Take a deep breath in and slowly exhale.

4. Slowly bring your knee and hand back to starting position. Repeat two more times.

5. Do the opposite side by raising your left knee and right hand off the floor. Repeat twice.

LEVEL UP:

You can make this exercise more challenging. When your knee and opposite hand are extended out, slowly bring that knee and opposite elbow together below you, exhaling as you do so. Do the same with the other side.

TAKE NOTE:

If this exercise causes you to lose your balance, keep both hands on the floor as you raise your leg. Alternatively, you can keep both knees on the floor as you raise your hand. Your core will strengthen over time.

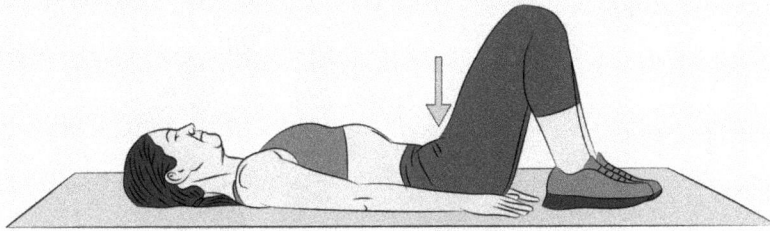

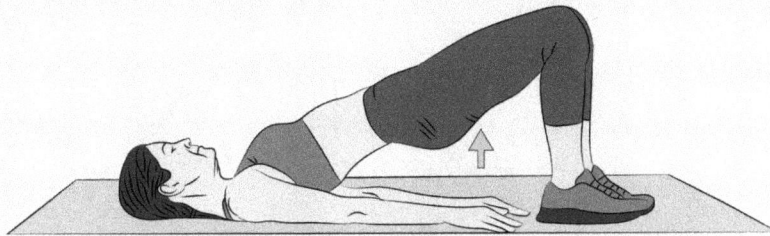

BRIDGE

TIME PER REP: 30 SECONDS | TOTAL TIME: 2 MINUTES

HOW TO:

1. Lie on your back on the mat. Bend your knees so that your feet are flat on the floor and knees are pointed towards the ceiling.

2. Place your feet about hip-width apart. Tighten your buttocks and abdominals as you slowly raise your hips straight up and off the floor. Your knees, hips, and shoulders should form a diagonal line.

3. Hold the raised position for two breaths in and out, then gently lower your hips back down to the floor.

4. Repeat three more times.

LEVEL UP:

To make this exercise more challenging, hold the raised bridge position for 30 seconds.

TAKE NOTE:

If you have any neck or spinal pain, check with your doctor and be extra cautious doing this exercise.

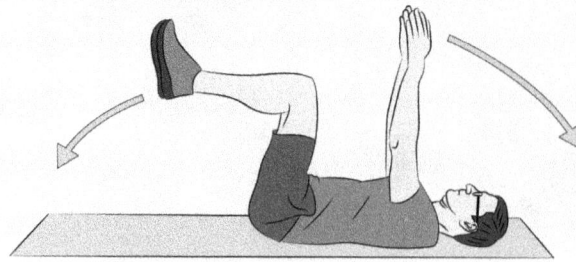

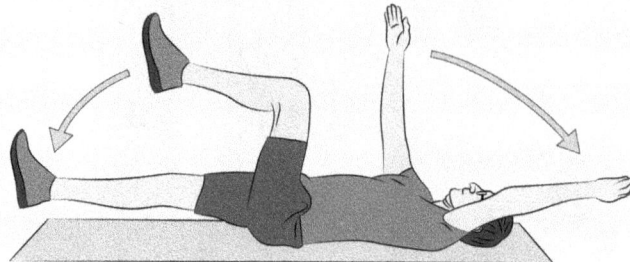

DEAD BUG

HOW TO:

1. Lie down with your back on the floor. Bend your knees and lift your feet off the floor so that your knees are directly over your hips.

2. Raise your feet so that your shins are parallel to the floor. Press the small of your back into the floor as you tighten your abdominals.

3. Lift both arms towards the ceiling with palms facing each other.

4. Keeping your knees bent, inhale and slowly lower your right foot until your toes touch the floor. Exhale and bring your foot back up to starting position.

5. Alternate doing the left foot and right foot, five times each.

LEVEL UP:

Once you are comfortable with this exercise, you can make it more challenging by adding the arms. As you lower one foot, also lower the opposite arm by reaching with your hand back above your head. Exhale as you return the foot and hand to the starting position. Alternate by doing the other hand and foot.

TAKE NOTE:

Don't arch your back while doing this exercise. Instead, keep your tummy firm and the small of your back pressed into the floor.

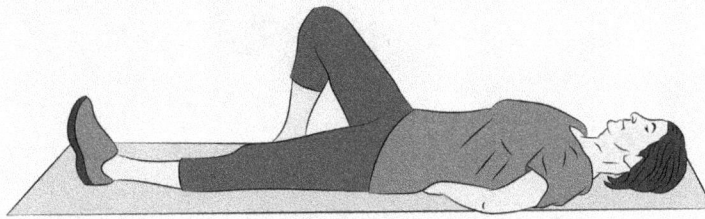

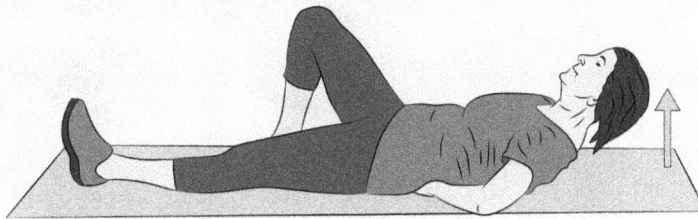

MODIFIED CURL UP

TIME PER REP: 15 SECONDS | TOTAL TIME: 2 MINUTES

HOW TO:

1. Lie down with your back on the mat. Bend both knees so that they are pointing to the ceiling and feet are flat on the floor.

2. Place your hands, palms down, between the floor and the small of your back. This will help protect your back.

3. Slowly straighten your right leg and extend your foot until the heel touches the floor. Keep your other leg bent.

4. Tighten your abdominals as you raise your head and shoulders slightly off the floor. Only raise them by one or two inches, this is not a large lift. Hold for five seconds and slowly lower back down.

5. Repeat the move three more times.

6. Switch legs. Straighten your left leg and extend your foot while keeping your other leg bent. Tighten your core as you raise your head and shoulders off the mat. Lower back down and repeat three more times.

LEVEL UP:

To make this more difficult, hold the lift for 10 seconds.

TAKE NOTE:

Be aware of your neck position while lifting your head and shoulders. Do not bend your neck forward to lift higher. Instead, keep your shoulders, neck, and head in a straight line.

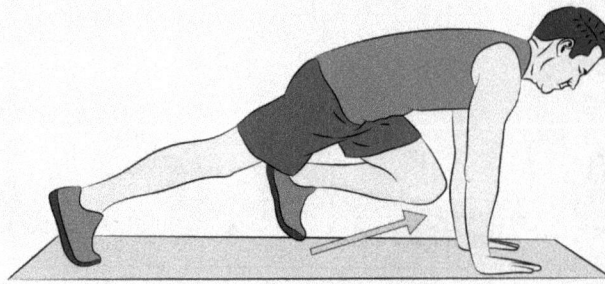

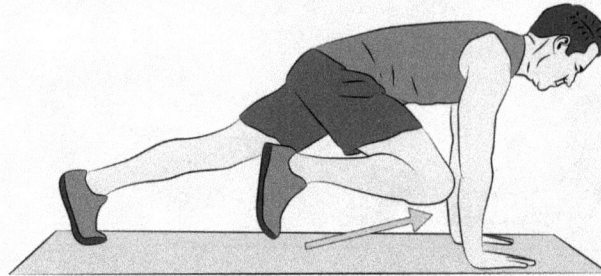

MOUNTAIN CLIMBER

TIME PER REP: 15 SECONDS | TOTAL TIME: 2 MINUTES

HOW TO:

1. Start from a kneeling position with your hands and knees on the mat.
2. Lift your knees from the mat and extend your legs straight behind you. Your hands should be directly under your shoulders and feet about hip-width apart with toes touching the mat.
3. From this plank position, tighten your abdominals and exhale as you bend your right knee and bring it up towards the middle of your chest. Inhale as you return your leg to the starting position.
4. Switch legs and exhale as you bend your left knee, bringing it towards the middle of your chest. Return your leg to the starting position.
5. Continue to do the mountain climbers, switching legs each time, for three more times on each leg.

LEVEL UP:

Add more repetitions as your core becomes stronger, working your way up to 10 or 12 times on each side.

TAKE NOTE:

Keep your eyes on the floor and don't let your head drop. Keep your neck long and in a straight line with your head and shoulders.

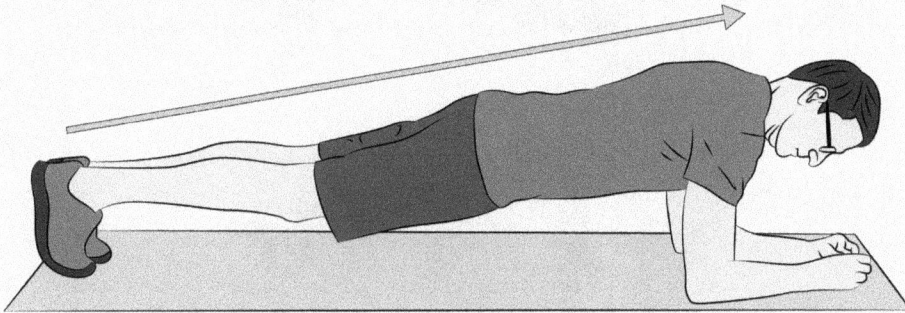

PLANK

TIME PER REP: 30 SECONDS | TOTAL TIME: 2 MINUTES

HOW TO:

1. Start from a kneeling position with your hands and knees on the mat.

2. Lift your knees from the mat and extend your legs out straight behind you. Your hands should be directly under your shoulders and feet about hip-width apart, with toes touching the mat.

3. Hold this plank position for 10 seconds. Lower knees to the floor and rest a few seconds. Repeat the plank three or four more times.

4. If this is too hard, try a modified plank. Instead of lifting both knees off the floor, only do one knee at a time.

LEVEL UP:

As you get stronger, hold the plank position for longer periods. Work up to 30 seconds, then one minute.

TAKE NOTE:

Pay attention to your lower back. Don't let it arch, but rather keep it in a straight line with your shoulders and hips.

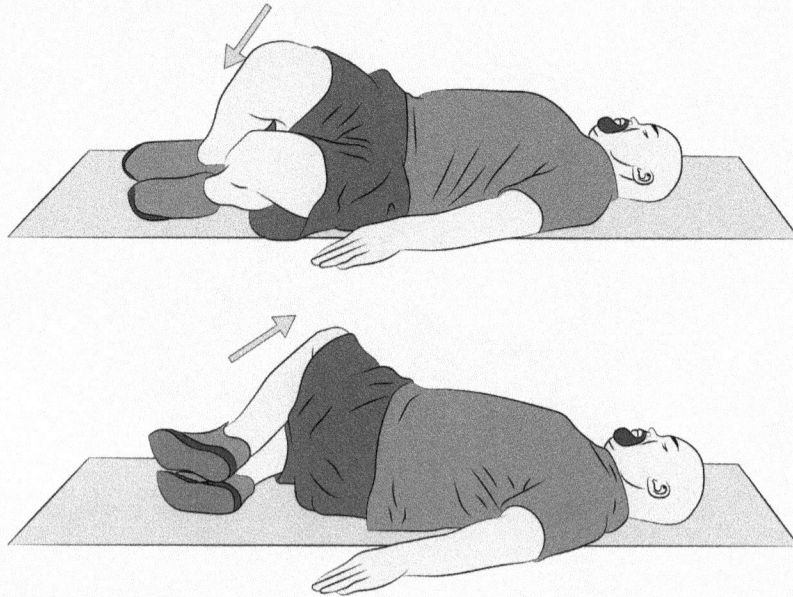

SEGMENTAL ROTATION

TIME PER REP: 20 SECONDS | TOTAL TIME: 2 MINUTES

HOW TO:

1. Lie down with your back on the floor.

2. Bend both knees so they are pointing to the ceiling, and both feet are on the floor. Extend both arms out from your sides, palms facing the floor.

3. Slowly lower both bent knees to the right side. Your upper body should face the ceiling, and only your lower body moves. You may be able to have your right knee lower all the way to the floor, but if you can't, that is okay. Only lower as far as you feel comfortable. It should not be painful.

4. Inhale, tighten your abdominals, and exhale as you raise both knees back to the starting position.

5. Doing the other side, lower both bent knees to the left as far as is comfortable. Bring both knees back to starting position.

6. Repeat the exercise on both sides three more times.

LEVEL UP:

As a variation, you can move your head and look in the opposite direction of your knees. If your knees are lowered to the right, rotate your head and look to the left. You will feel a gentle stretch on the right side of your neck. When your knees are lowered to the left, look right.

TAKE NOTE:

Keep both shoulders firmly planted on the mat. Neither shoulder should be lifting at any time during the rotation. If it does, you are rotating too far.

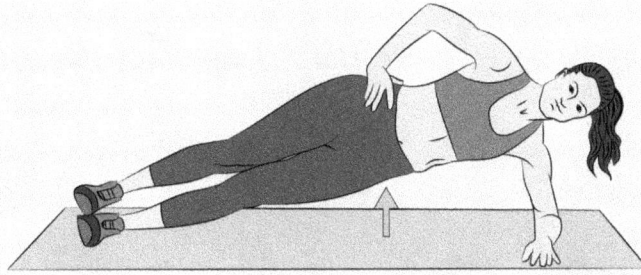

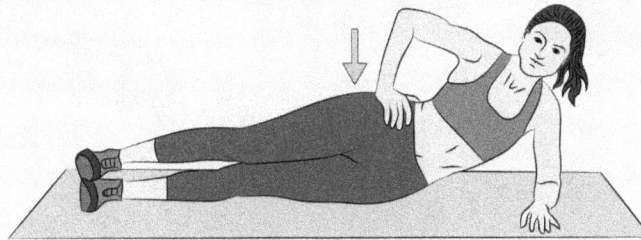

SIDE PLANK

HOW TO:

1. Lie on the floor on your right side. Extend your legs, so they are straight, with hips stacked one on top of the other.

2. Bring your right arm under you. Prop up your upper body by placing your right forearm on the floor directly under your right shoulder. Be sure your right forearm and hand are placed on the floor for support.

3. Tighten your core and raise your hips up and off the floor. Your feet, knees, hips, and shoulders should form a straight diagonal line. Breathing normally, hold for five seconds.

4. Slowly lower hip back down to the floor. Rest a few seconds, then repeat the side plank three more times.

5. Switch to your left side. Doing the same thing on this side, extend your legs and bring your left arm under you. Raise your hips off the floor to form a diagonal line and hold for five seconds. Lower and repeat three more times.

6. If this exercise is too hard, try doing it with your bottom leg bent and resting on the floor instead.

LEVEL UP:

Once five seconds is easy for you, increase your time to 10 or 20 seconds on each side. To make this exercise even more challenging, you can do it with your bottom hand on the floor and your arm fully extended. You will be supporting yourself with your hand rather than your forearm.

TAKE NOTE:

Don't let your hips droop down. Keep the diagonal line from your feet, knees, hips, and shoulders.

27

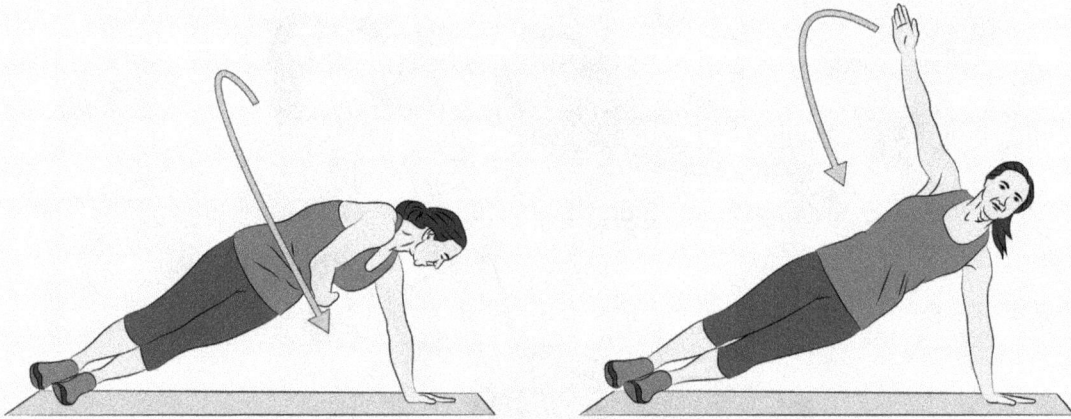

SIDE PLANK WITH ROTATION

TIME PER REP: 20 SECONDS | TOTAL TIME: 2 MINUTES

HOW TO:

1. Get into a side plank position, lying on your right side with legs extended, hips stacked, and right forearm on the floor supporting you.
2. Tighten your core muscles as you lift your hips off the floor.
3. Extend your left arm up towards the ceiling and inhale.
4. Exhale and bring your left arm down and under your right ribs.
5. Return your left arm up and extend it towards the ceiling.
6. Slowly lower your hips to the floor. Repeat the sequence three more times.
7. Switch sides by lying on your left side. Lift your hips off the floor and now extend your right arm to the ceiling, bring it down under your left ribs, and extend up again. Lower your hips and repeat three more times.

LEVEL UP:

You can change the intensity of this exercise. To make it easier, keep your bottom leg bent and resting on the floor. To make it more challenging, support yourself with your hand and a straight arm instead of your forearm.

TAKE NOTE:

Keep your gaze straight ahead in front of you. If your balance is good, your eyes and head can follow your moving arm as it goes underneath you.

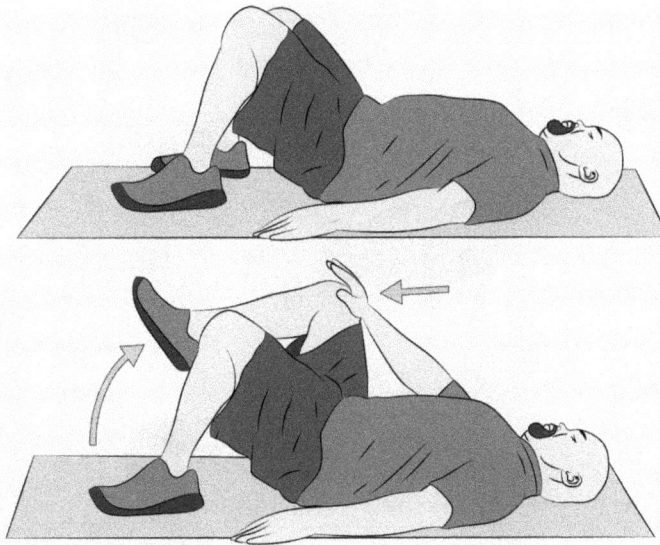

SINGLE-LEG ABDOMINAL PRESS

TIME PER REP: 15 SECONDS | TOTAL TIME: 2 MINUTES

HOW TO:

1. Lie on the mat on your back. Bend both knees so that they are pointing towards the ceiling, and your feet are flat on the floor.

2. Raise your right leg and foot so that your shin is parallel to the floor. Your knee should be at a 90-degree angle.

3. Tighten your abdominals as you place your right hand on your right knee and try to press it away from you. At the same time, have your right knee resist against your hand. Hold for five seconds, then lower your leg to the starting position. Repeat on this side three more times.

4. Switch legs. Raise your left leg and foot, forming a 90-degree angle. With your left hand, press your left knee away from you while trying to resist with your knee. Repeat on this side three more times.

LEVEL UP:

To make this more challenging, raise both knees simultaneously. Press both hands against both knees as they resist.

TAKE NOTE:

Keep your back in a neutral position. Neither arch your lower back nor press it into the floor.

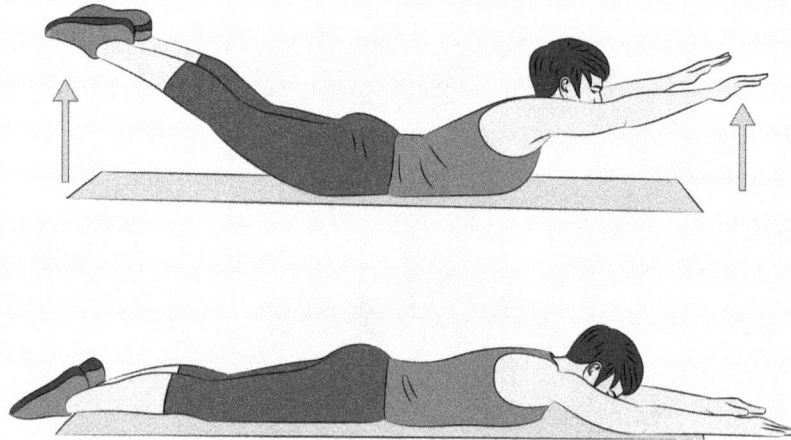

SUPERMAN

HOW TO:

1. Lie on the floor, face down, with arms overhead and legs extended out straight.

2. Inhale, tighten your core muscles, and while exhaling, simultaneously raise your chest, arms, and legs off the floor a few inches. Hold the position for five seconds, then slowly lower back down to the floor. Repeat six times.

3. To make this exercise easier, you can choose to raise only your chest and arms off the floor. Or raise only your legs off the floor.

LEVEL UP:

Make this exercise more challenging by making small flutter or paddling motions while your arms and legs are lifted.

TAKE NOTE:

If your hips need extra support, place a folded towel under them. You can also place one under your forehead.

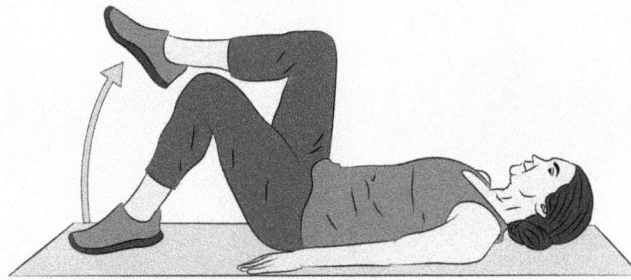

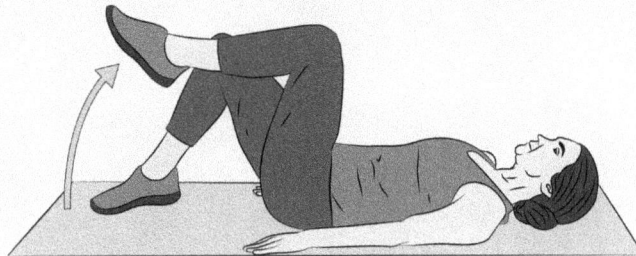

SUPINE TOE TAPS

TIME PER REP: 15 SECONDS | TOTAL TIME: 2 MINUTES

HOW TO:

1. Lie down with your back on a mat. Bend your knees so they face the ceiling and feet are flat on the mat. Rest arms at your side with palms facing down.

2. Slowly raise both feet up off the mat so that your shins are now parallel to the floor and knees are at a 90-degree angle.

3. Keeping your right knee bent, lower your right foot to the floor until your toes touch. Bring the foot back up.

4. Now do the same with your left foot, tapping the floor with your left toes and bringing it back up.

5. Alternate feet, doing a total of four toe taps per foot.

LEVEL UP:

Increase the number of toe taps as your core gets stronger. To make this harder, do both feet at the same time.

TAKE NOTE:

Don't arch your back while performing this exercise. If your lower back needs extra support, place your hands or a small, folded towel under the small of your back.

Chapter 4:
Seated Core Exercises

Life isn't about finding yourself.
Life is about creating yourself.

—George Bernard Shaw

You may be surprised to learn that seated exercises are an effective way to strengthen your core. Seated exercising is a low-impact and safe way to work your core and get in some cardio movement and strength training. If you have suffered from a stroke, fall, or another challenge that has weakened your core, seated exercises are a smart way to regain your strength and balance. It also lessens the likelihood of falling. Seated exercises are perfect for those who find it challenging to get down and up from the floor, those who are disabled and require a wheelchair, or those who have balance and stability issues. These seated exercises can help you regain and maintain a strong core and will help build your confidence and abilities to perform daily tasks.

In this chapter, we will look at twelve of the best seated exercises for your core. For these seated exercises, it is recommended to sit in a sturdy, straight-backed chair with no arms. If you need extra stability, place the chair near a table or low counter that you can place your hand upon if required.

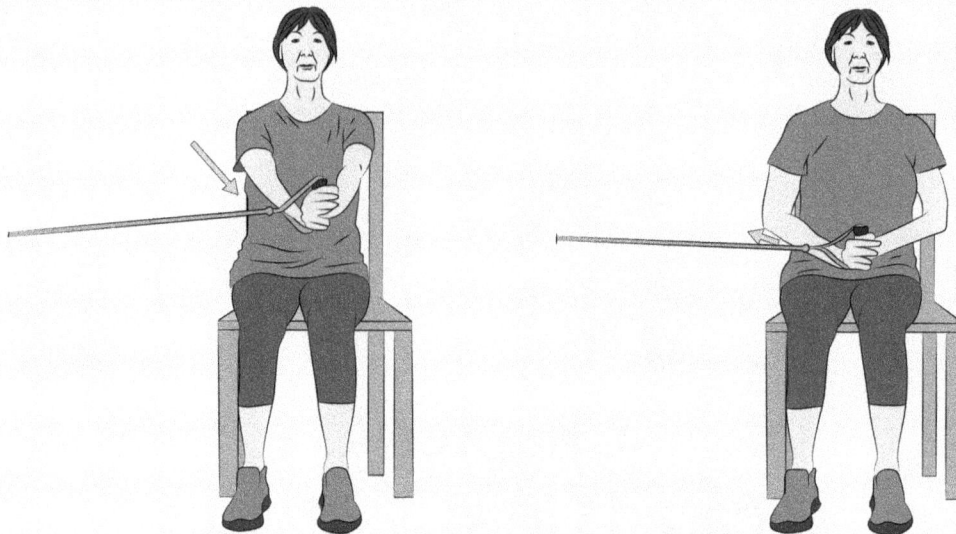

BAND EXTENSION

HOW TO:

1. Loop a resistance band around the back of a sturdy chair.

2. Sit down in the chair. Place your hands in the handles and loop the band around your hands until the band is taut when your hands are resting in your lap.

3. Sit up tall with your feet flat on the floor. With arms bent, lift both hands to the same height as your belly button.

4. Tighten your core muscles. Push your hands out straight in front of you until your arms are fully extended. You should feel resistance from the band. Hold for five seconds, then bend arms and return your hands to your lap.

5. Repeat seven more times.

LEVEL UP:

If you don't have a resistance band, you can use three-pound weights in each hand instead. There won't be resistance, but your core muscles will still be exercised.

TAKE NOTE:

Don't slouch or hunch up while doing this exercise. Sit up tall and keep your shoulders relaxed and down.

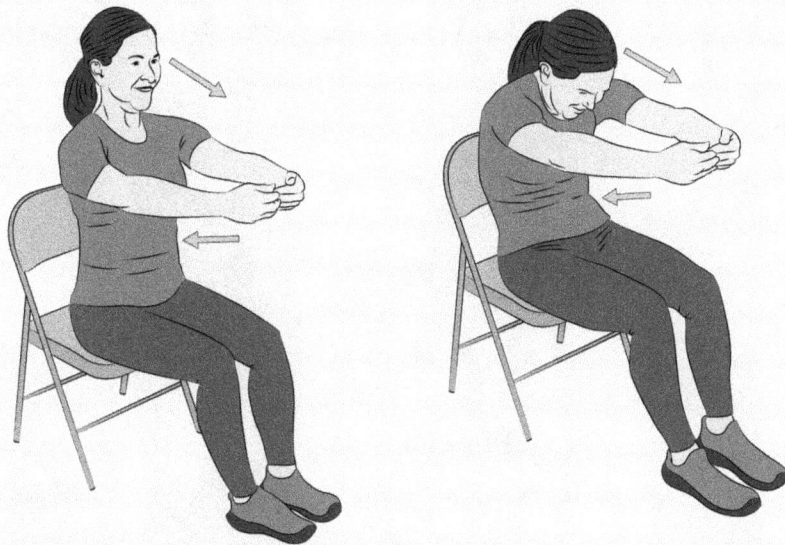

HALF ROLLBACKS

TIME PER REP: 15 SECONDS | TOTAL TIME: 2 MINUTES

HOW TO:

1. Sit erect in a chair with your feet flat on the floor and knees bent.
2. Lift both arms out in front of you with your elbows bent, fingertips touching, and palms facing towards you.
3. Slowly round your shoulders and upper back as you contract your abdominals and look down at your thighs. Hold for five seconds, then slowly roll back up. Once returned to the starting position, reset your shoulders by shrugging them up, back, and down.
4. Repeat the exercise seven more times.

LEVEL UP:

You can make this slightly more difficult. Instead of having your feet flat on the floor while seated, raise your heels so that only your toes are touching the floor.

TAKE NOTE:

It's natural to hold your breath while performing this exercise. Remember to breathe normally.

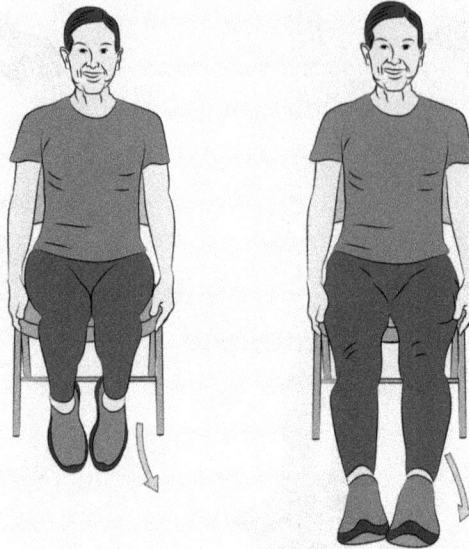

LEG TAPS

HOW TO:

1. Sit upright in a chair or on a bench with your knees bent. Sit closer towards the edge but with your buttocks still on the seat.

2. With feet flat on the floor, place your hands on the seat of the chair for support.

3. Extend both legs out straight in front of you with feet still touching the floor. Tighten up your abdominals as you lift both feet off the floor a few inches. Hold for five seconds and slowly lower back down to the floor.

4. Repeat three more times.

LEVEL UP:

To increase the difficulty, you can hold your feet off the floor for 10 seconds, then 20 seconds.

TAKE NOTE:

Be sure not to hunch up your shoulders or lean too far back when you raise your legs up. Try to maintain an upright position.

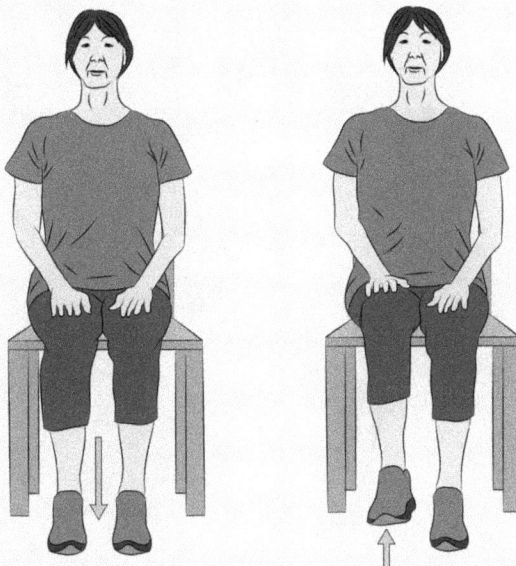

RESISTED KNEE LIFT

TIME PER REP: 15 SECONDS | TOTAL TIME: 2 MINUTES

HOW TO:

1. With your knees bent, sit up tall in a chair with your feet flat on the floor.
2. Place your hands on your thighs, palms down.
3. Keeping your right knee bent, raise your thigh a few inches off the chair. At the same time, press your right hand down on your thigh to resist it. Tighten your abs and hold for five seconds. Lower your leg back down.
4. Switching legs, raise your left thigh off the chair while pressing your left hand down upon it. Hold for five seconds and then lower.
5. Repeat the exercise three more times.

LEVEL UP:

You can make this harder by lifting both legs at the same time while pressing down on them with both hands.

TAKE NOTE:

Maintain good posture while doing this move.

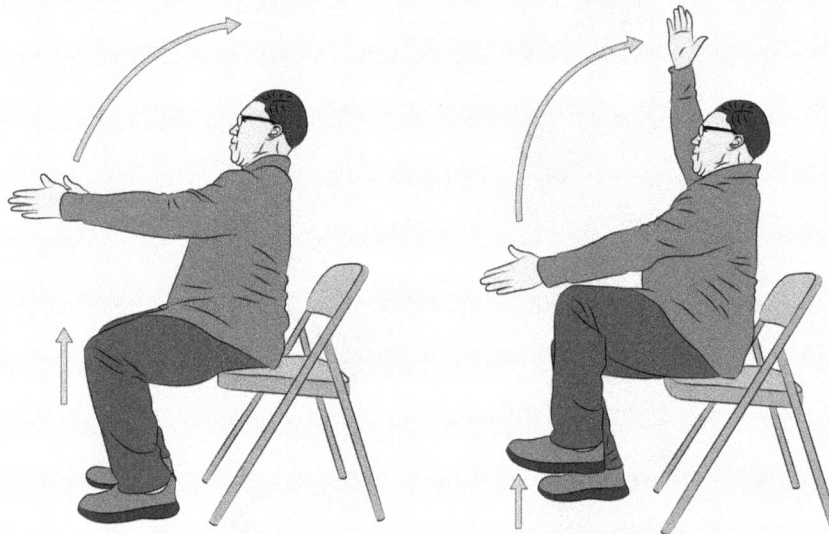

SEATED DEAD BUG

TIME PER REP: 10 SECONDS | TOTAL TIME: 2 MINUTES

HOW TO:

1. Sit erect in a chair. Your knees should be bent and your feet flat on the floor.
2. Raise both arms straight out in front of you.
3. Inhale. As you exhale, tighten your tummy and lift your right arm up above your head. Bring your arm back down so it is straight out in front of you.
4. Switch arms. This time lift your left arm above your head while tightening your abs. Return the arm to the starting position.
5. Repeat on both arms five more times.

LEVEL UP:

To increase the difficulty, raise the opposite foot off the floor as you bring your arm up above your head.

TAKE NOTE:

It's tempting to do this exercise quickly and wind up pumping your arms up and down. Remember to move through the exercise slowly and deliberately while keeping your tummy tightened.

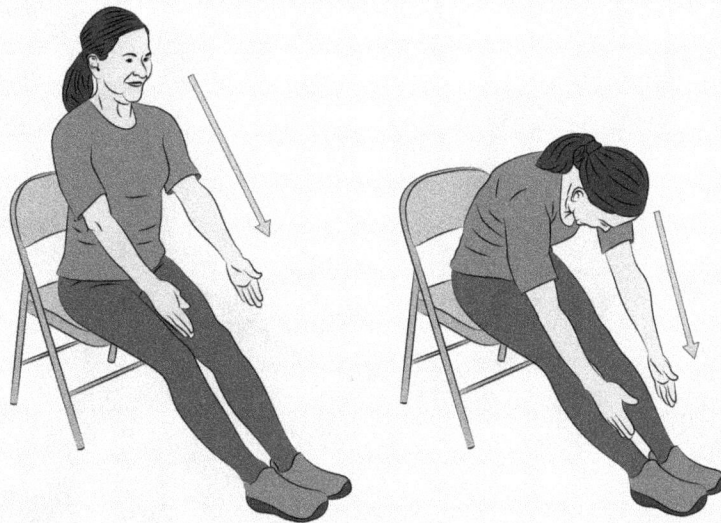

SEATED FORWARD ROLL-UP

TIME PER REP: 15 SECONDS | TOTAL TIME: 2 MINUTES

HOW TO:

1. Sit up tall in a chair. Extend both legs out in front of you with your heels on the floor and toes pointed to the ceiling.
2. Raise your arms straight out in front of you.
3. Tuck your chin in towards your chest as you roll forward with your arms extended. Your hands should be reaching towards your toes.
4. Tighten your abs and slowly roll back up to the starting position.
5. Repeat the exercise seven more times.

LEVEL UP:

Once you are comfortable with this exercise, you can increase the difficulty. Take twice as long to roll back up as you did to roll down.

TAKE NOTE:

Be sure to do these moves slowly, so you don't use any momentum as you roll down or up.

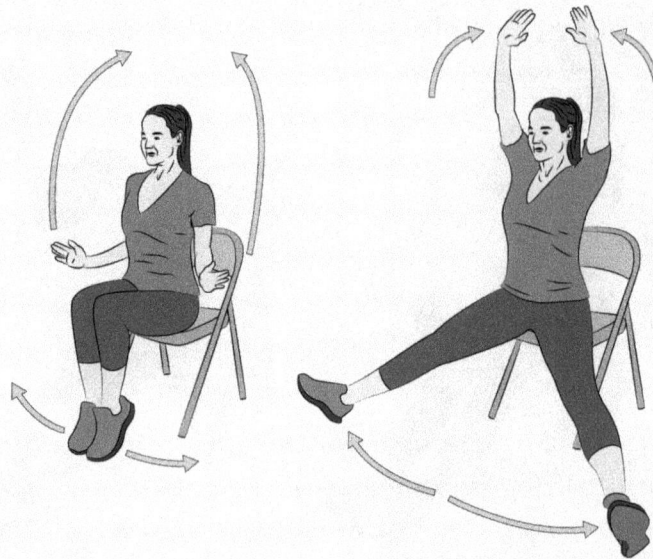

SEATED JUMPING JACKS

TIME PER REP: 10 SECONDS | TOTAL TIME: 1 MINUTE

HOW TO:

1. Sit erect in a chair with your knees bent. Have your feet on the floor but with your heels slightly lifted. Hands are down on either side of you.

2. Tighten your abs as you raise both hands up above your head. Simultaneously lift both feet off the floor and out to the sides like you would for a standing jumping jack. Bring hands and feet back to starting position.

3. Repeat the exercise five more times.

4. If you find this to be too hard, do the seated jumping jacks one side at a time. Instead of lifting both arms and both legs, just do the left arm and left leg. Switch to the other leg and repeat.

LEVEL UP:

This exercise can also count as cardio when 30 or more jumping jacks are done. For those who have knee or hip pain, this is a low-impact way to do jumping jacks.

TAKE NOTE:

Don't allow your neck to crane forward or your upper back to hunch while completing these moves. Keep your neck and upper back neutral and relaxed.

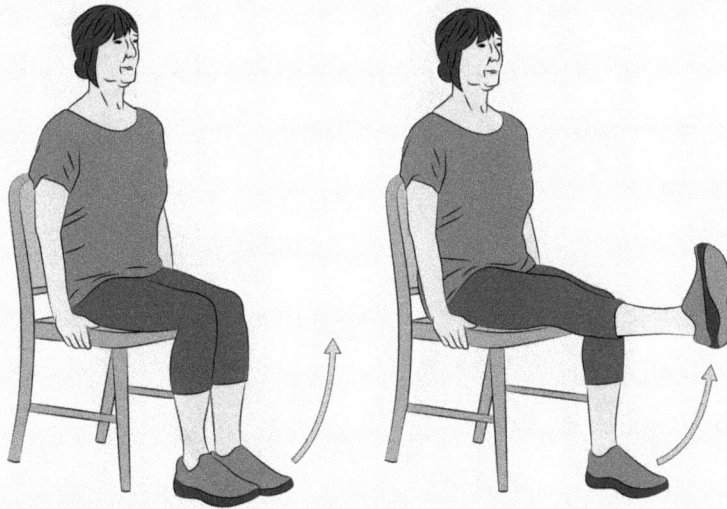

SEATED LEG LIFT

HOW TO:

1. With both feet flat on the floor, sit in a chair with your knees bent. Place your hands on either side of the chair seat for support.

2. Straighten your right leg while keeping your foot on the floor. Tighten your tummy as you raise your right foot off the floor until it is parallel to the floor, if possible. Hold the position for five seconds, then slowly lower your foot back to the floor.

3. Reset by sitting with both knees bent. Switch to the other side by straightening your left leg. Raise your left foot and hold for five seconds before lowering back down.

4. Repeat each leg three more times.

LEVEL UP:

As a variation, you can concentrate on one leg at a time. Do all six reps with one leg before switching to the other instead of alternating legs.

TAKE NOTE:

Be sure not to slouch or round your back as you lift your leg.

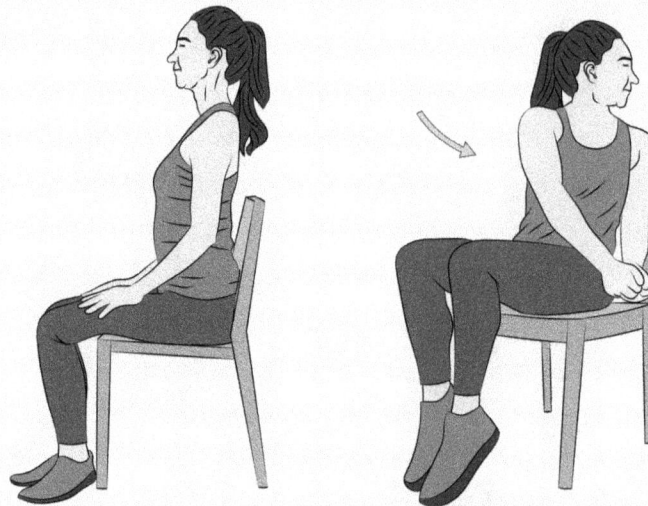

SEATED RUSSIAN TWIST

TIME PER REP: 15 SECONDS | TOTAL TIME: 2 MINUTES

HOW TO:

1. Sit up tall in a chair. Your knees should be bent and your feet on the floor with your heels slightly lifted.

2. Bend your elbows at a 90-degree angle with your hands in front of you. Clasp your hands together, interlocking your fingers.

3. Tighten your abs as you move your clasped hands to the outside of your right leg, then slowly move your hands to the outside of your left leg. Allow your eyes, head, and shoulders to follow the movement of your hands. Breathe normally throughout.

4. Repeat the exercise seven more times.

LEVEL UP:

Increase the difficulty by lifting your feet completely off the floor as you twist from side to side.

TAKE NOTE:

This should be a slow, continuous movement as you move your hands from side to side. Take care not to jerk your hands over as you change sides.

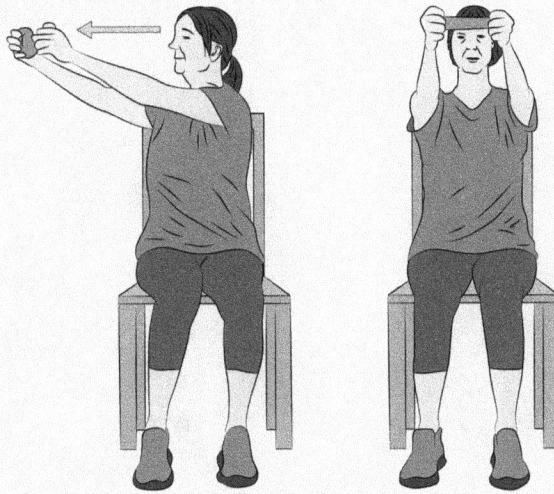

SEATED TWIST

TIME PER REP: 20 SECONDS | TOTAL TIME: 2 MINUTES

HOW TO:

1. Sit in a chair with your feet flat on the floor.
2. Raise your arms and hands straight out in front of you so that your hands are at eye level.
3. Tighten your core as you move your hands and arms to the right while gently twisting your torso. Hands should still be at eye level. Hold the twist for five seconds. The rotation should stem from your midsection, not just your shoulders. Slowly return to starting position with arms straight ahead.
4. Now twist to the other side by bringing your arms to the left while twisting your midsection. Hold for five seconds before returning to the starting position.
5. Repeat the exercise five more times.

LEVEL UP:

To make this exercise more challenging, hold a three to five-pound weight while doing the twists.

TAKE NOTE:

Check with your doctor before doing this or any twisting exercise if you have osteoporosis or have recently had back surgery.

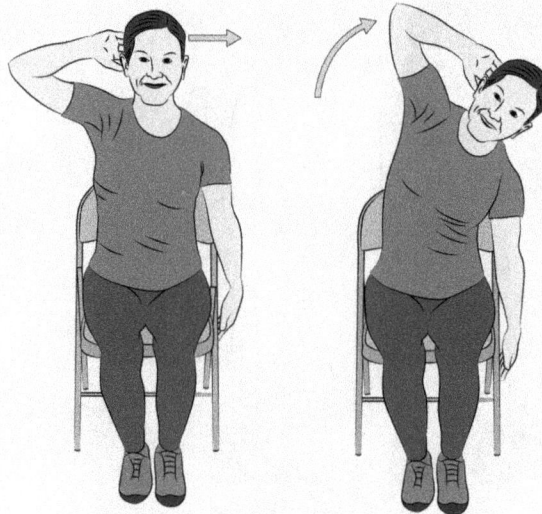

SIDE BENDS

TIME PER REP: 15 SECONDS | TOTAL TIME: 1 MINUTE

HOW TO:

1. Sit in a chair and maintain good posture. Knees should be bent, and feet flat on the floor. Let your arms hang down on either side of your body.

2. Take a breath in and as you exhale, lower your right arm towards the floor as you bend sideways at the waist. Using your core muscles, slowly come back up to the starting position.

3. Switch to the other side by lowering your left arm to the floor as you exhale and bend sideways to the left. Slowly return to the starting position.

4. Repeat exercise five more times.

LEVEL UP:

Add some resistResisted Knee Liftance by holding three-pound weights in each hand as you do the side bends.

TAKE NOTE:

Take care that your chest is facing forward as you bend at the waist. Don't allow your chest to twist and face the floor.

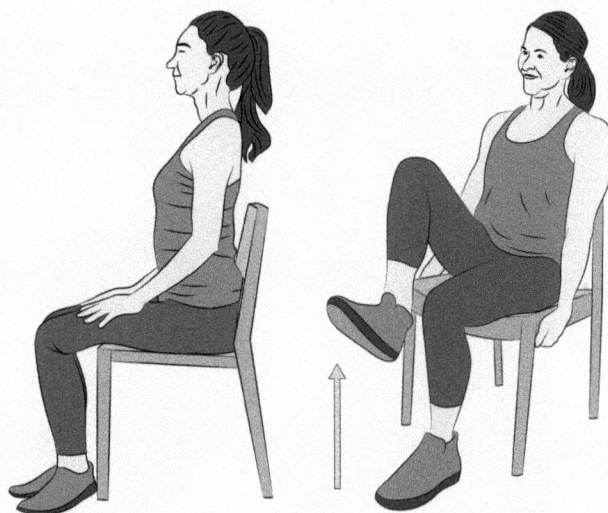

SINGLE KNEE TUCK

TIME PER REP: 20 SECONDS | TOTAL TIME: 2 MINUTES

HOW TO:

1. Sit up tall. Come closer to the edge of the chair but still have both buttocks fully on the seat. Be sure your knees are bent, and feet are flat on the floor.

2. Grip the sides of the seat with both hands for support.

3. Keeping your knee bent, raise your right knee until it is higher than your hip, if possible. Hold it up for five seconds as you keep your abs tight. Lower your leg back down to the starting position.

4. Switch legs, this time lifting your left knee and holding for five seconds. Lower the leg back down.

5. Repeat five more times.

LEVEL UP:

To make this more challenging, lift both knees at the same time.

TAKE NOTE:

Be sure not to lean back as you lift your knees. Maintain an upright posture.

Chapter 5:
Standing Core Exercises

Aging gracefully means being flexible, being open, allowing change, enjoying change and loving yourself.

—Wendy Whelan

Can you exercise your core while you are standing? You can! Performing core exercises from a standing position provides a change from how core exercises are traditionally done and provides some fresh moves for core muscle training. Surprising your muscles causes them to be stimulated and grow due to the change in position and type of exercise. You can keep your muscles guessing by not doing the same old same old. Standing exercises require a little more balance and stability on your feet. Use a sturdy chair or nearby countertop for extra support.

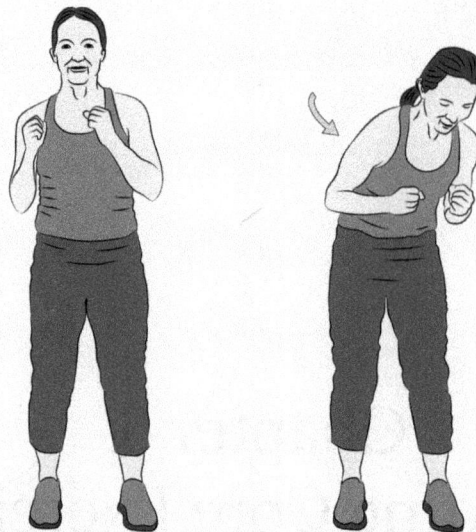

CORE ROTATION

HOW TO:

1. Stand up tall. Have your knees slightly bent and your feet hip-width distance apart and flat on the floor.
2. Bend your arms at the elbows to form a 90-degree angle with your hands out in front of you.
3. Keeping your abdominals tight, bend your torso over to the right, bend forward, then bend to the left. This should be a smooth arc going from the right side to the left side.
4. Do the same thing but going in the other direction. Bend your torso over to the left, forward, and right in a smooth movement while keeping your abs tight.
5. Repeat five more times.

LEVEL UP:

To add difficulty to this move, hold a three or five-pound weight with both hands.

TAKE NOTE:

It's easy to hold your breath as you concentrate on your abs. Keep breathing normally throughout this exercise.

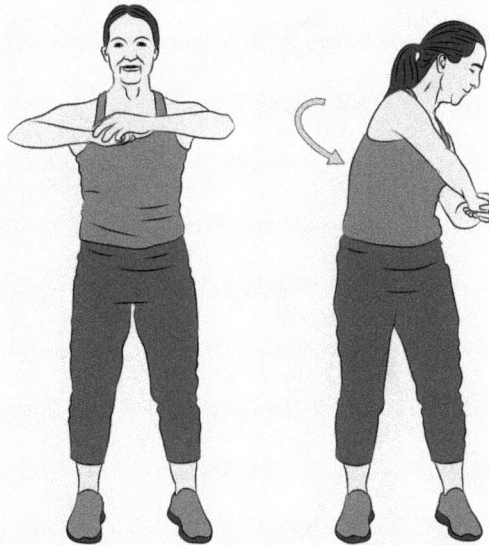

FIGURE 8 ROW

TIME PER REP: 10 SECONDS | TOTAL TIME: 1 MINUTE

HOW TO:

1. Stand comfortably with feet hip-width distance apart and flat on the floor. Knees can be slightly bent.

2. Raise both arms and bend at your elbows. Place one hand under the opposite elbow and let the other hand rest on top of the other elbow. Your forearms should be resting one on top of the other at chest height.

3. Keep your posture upright as you tighten your ab muscles and move your right elbow down towards your right hip. Bring your right elbow up to shoulder height.

4. Work the other side by moving your left elbow down to your left hip, then up to shoulder height. Your elbows should be drawing a figure-eight in the air in front of you.

5. Repeat the move, alternating side, five more times.

LEVEL UP:

If you have shoulder pain or it is difficult for you to stack one forearm on top of the other, an option is to hold your hands out in front of you with elbows at a 90-degree angle. Make a fist with both hands with palms down and knuckles up. Do the figure-eight motion now. It will mimic paddling a canoe, minus the oar.

TAKE NOTE:

Don't let your torso hunch over too far to the right or left. Maintain an upright posture and let your abs do the work.

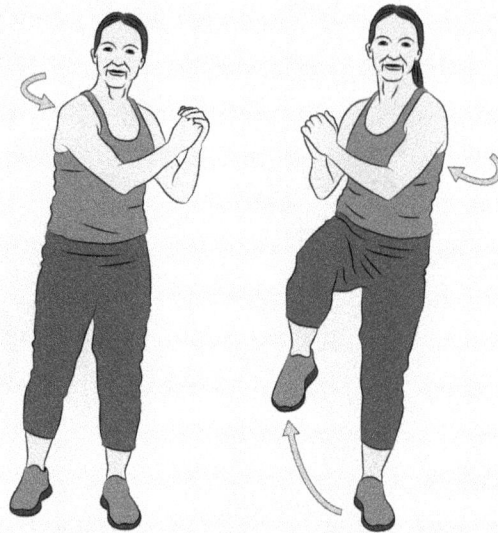

KNEE ROTATION

TIME PER REP: 10 SECONDS | TOTAL TIME: 2 MINUTES

HOW TO:

1. Stand up tall with both feet flat on the floor and hip-width distance apart.
2. Clasp both hands together in front of you with elbows bent at a 90-degree angle.
3. Bring your hands over to the right side of your waist and let your torso twist to the right.
4. Now, bring your hands to the left side and twist your torso to the left. Simultaneously, lift your left knee and foot as your torso twists to the left.
5. Bring your left knee down as you twist back to the right side.
6. Repeat this same side five more times.
7. Switch sides by starting with your hands over on the left side of your waist and twisting your torso to the left. As you bring your hands over the right and twist to the right, raise your right knee. Repeat on this side five more times.

LEVEL UP:

If you can't lift your entire foot off the floor without losing your balance, you can modify this move by just lifting your heel off the floor while keeping your toes connected to the floor.

TAKE NOTE:

Remember to keep your core muscles engaged throughout this exercise; otherwise, you are just twisting!

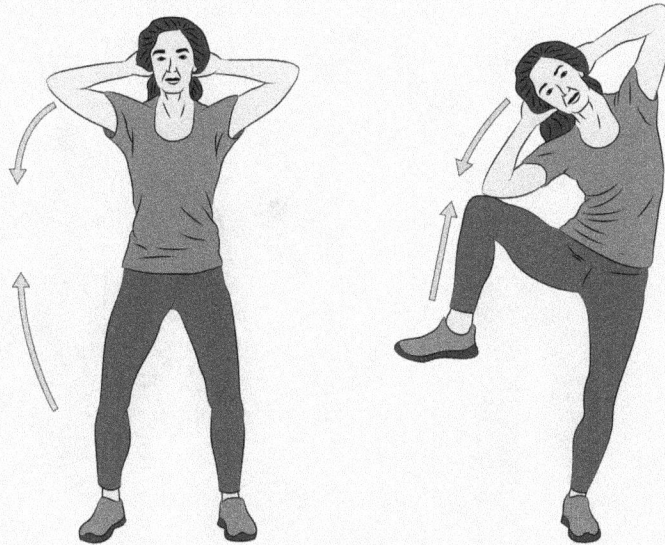

KNEE TUCK EXTENSION

TIME PER REP: 10 SECONDS | TOTAL TIME: 2 MINUTES

HOW TO:

1. Stand up tall with feet hip-width distance apart. If you need a sturdy chair or countertop to hold on to for balance, stand next to that.

2. Stretch your right arm up overhead and inhale. As you exhale, bend your arm and bring your elbow down. At the same time, raise your right knee and try to have your elbow and knee touch. Your left hand can rest on your waist or on a chair.

3. Repeat five more times.

4. Switch sides. Now stretch your left arm overhead and bring your left elbow down as you bring your left knee up to meet it. Repeat five more times on this side.

LEVEL UP:

To increase the difficulty, bend both arms and place your hands behind your head. Facing straight ahead, bend your torso to the right as you bring your right elbow and knee towards each other. Do the same thing on the left.

TAKE NOTE:

You are bringing your elbow and knee towards each other. It's okay if they don't touch.

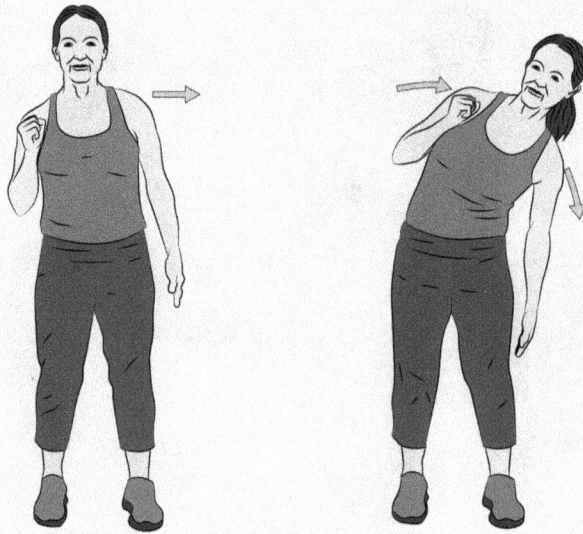

STANDING SIDE BENDS

TIME PER REP: 10 SECONDS | TOTAL TIME: 2 MINUTES

HOW TO:

1. Stand erect with your feet at hip-width distance apart and feet flat on the floor.

2. Bend your left arm at the elbow with your left hand out in front of you so that your left elbow forms a 90-degree angle. Let your right arm hang straight down at your right side.

3. Keeping your chest and head looking straight ahead, tighten your abs as you bend your torso to the right so that your right-hand slides down your right side towards your right knee. Return to the starting position. Repeat five more times.

4. Switch sides by bending your right elbow and having your left arm down by your side. Bend your torso to the left and allow your left hand to slide down your left side. Return to the starting position, then repeat five more times.

LEVEL UP:

Adding two or three-pound hand weights will make this exercise more challenging. Take care not to add too heavy of a weight.

TAKE NOTE:

Don't let your chest collapse as you bend to the side. Keep your chest out and facing straight ahead.

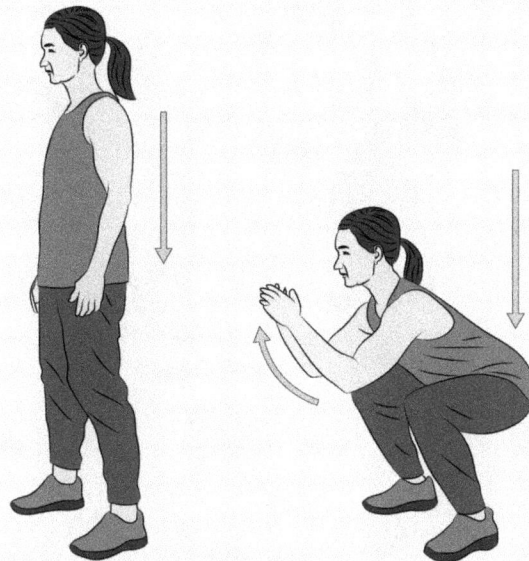

SQUAT

HOW TO:

1. Stand with your feet hip-width distance apart.
2. Raise both arms straight out in front of you as you bend your knees.
3. Squat as low as is comfortable and hold for five seconds. Return to standing.
4. Repeat the exercise five more times.

LEVEL UP:

You can make this more challenging by doing more squats. Try to do 10 in a row, then 20, and increase from there.

TAKE NOTE:

Squats work on your core muscles in your lower back, pelvis, and glutes. If you have balancing issues, be sure to hold on to a sturdy chair or countertop.

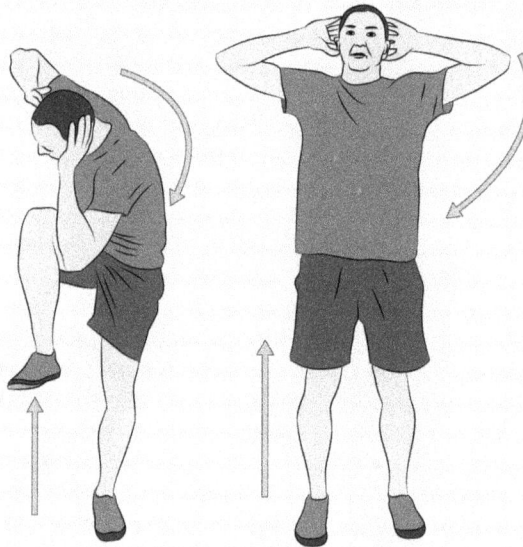

STANDING BICYCLE CRUNCH

HOW TO:

1. Stand up tall with feet hip-width distance apart and knees slightly bent.
2. Have a sturdy chair or countertop next to you for balance. Bend your right arm and place your right hand behind your head.
3. Bend your left knee and lift your left foot off the floor. Twist your torso to bring your right elbow towards your raised left knee. Return to the starting position.
4. Repeat the exercise on this side five more times.
5. Switch sides. Place your left hand behind your head and lift your right foot off the floor. Twist to the right as you bring your left elbow to your right knee. Repeat five times.

LEVEL UP:

If you don't have stability challenges, try doing this without holding on to anything. Place both hands behind your head as you do the standing crunches, alternating from one knee to the other.

TAKE NOTE:

Be sure you are not pulling on your neck or bending it too far forward as you move through your crunches.

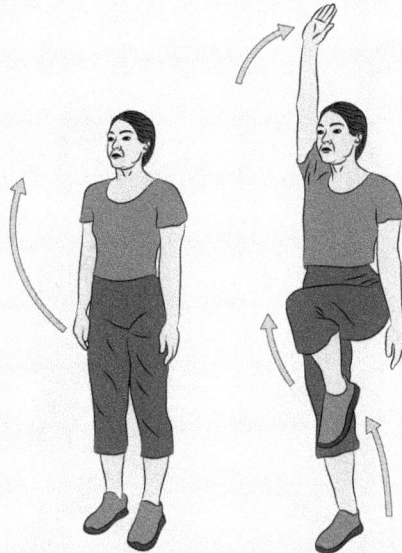

STANDING BIRD DOG

TIME PER REP: 10 SECONDS | TOTAL TIME: 2 MINUTES

HOW TO:

1. Stand up tall with your feet hip-width distance apart, and arms by your sides.

2. Stand next to a sturdy chair or countertop to hold on to for balance. Raise your right hand straight above your head while at the same time raising your left knee and left foot off the floor. Hold this pose for five seconds, then return to the starting position.

3. Repeat this side five more times.

4. Switch sides by raising your left hand above your head while raising the opposite knee. Repeat five more times.

LEVEL UP:

Add a balance challenge to this exercise by not holding on to anything.

TAKE NOTE:

Moving slowly through this exercise and contracting your core muscles will ensure that you are working them.

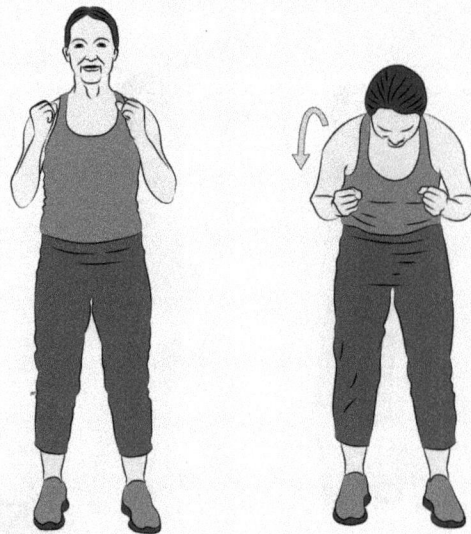

STANDING CRUNCH

HOW TO:

1. Stand with feet about hip-width distance apart and knees slightly bent.
2. Bend your elbows so that your hands are out in front of you and elbows are at a 90-degree angle.
3. Inhale. As you exhale, tighten your core, and slowly bend forward at the waist. Bend forward as far as you can comfortably, but don't go lower than your belly button. Slowly return to a standing position.
4. Repeat five more times.

LEVEL UP:

As a variation, you can raise your hands and place them behind your head as you would for regular sit-ups. Be sure not to pull on your neck.

TAKE NOTE:

Keep your shoulders relaxed as you move through this exercise. Don't allow them to hunch up.

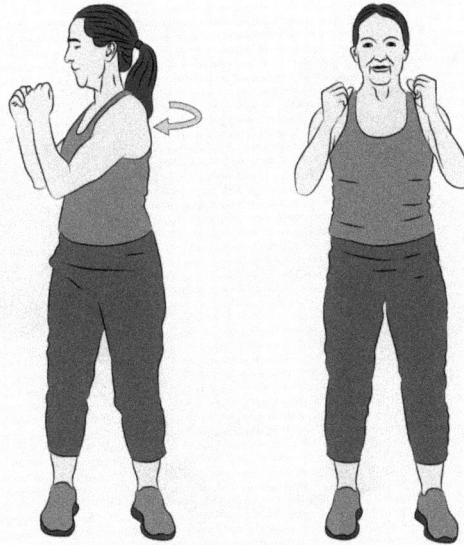

STANDING TWIST

TIME PER REP: 10 SECONDS | TOTAL TIME: 1 MINUTE

HOW TO:

1. With feet about hip-width distance apart and feet flat on the floor, stand up tall.
2. Bend your arms at the elbow with your hands in front of you so that elbows form a 90-degree angle.
3. Keeping your hips straight ahead, tighten your abs and twist your torso and arms turning to the right.
4. Come back to the starting point and twist your torso and arms turning to the left.
5. Repeat the moves five more times.

LEVEL UP:

To increase the difficulty, hold a two or three-pound weight in each hand.

TAKE NOTE:

Don't swing from side to side using momentum. This should be a slow, deliberate twist from the waist up. Keep your feet stationary.

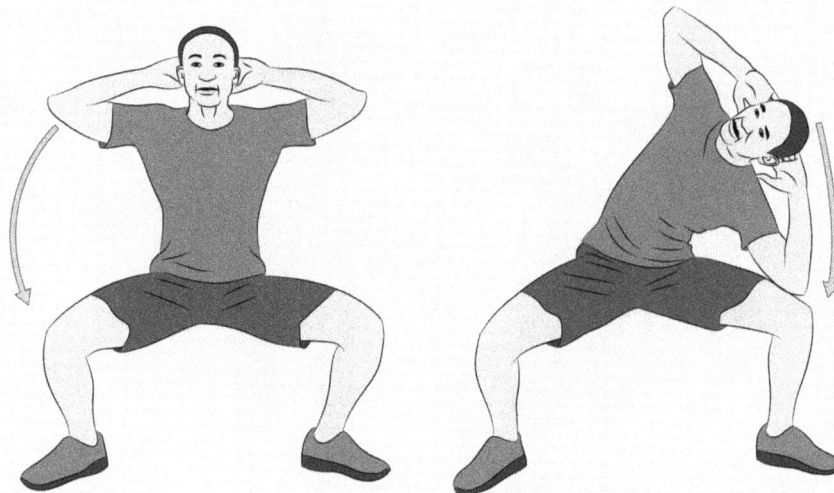

WIDE SIDE CRUNCH

TIME PER REP: 10 SECONDS | TOTAL TIME: 2 MINUTES

HOW TO:

1. Stand with your feet wide apart, and toes slightly pointed out. Bend your knees as far as is comfortable or until thighs are almost parallel with the floor.

2. Bend both arms and place your hands behind your head.

3. Keep your chest facing straight ahead, bend your torso and upper body over to the right. Your right elbow should be reaching down towards your right thigh. Return to center. Repeat five more times.

4. Now bend your torso and upper body over to the left with your left elbow pointing down towards your left thigh. Return to center and repeat five more times.

LEVEL UP:

Instead of doing one side at a time, alternate bending to the right and then to the left.

TAKE NOTE:

Don't pull on your neck or hunch forward as you do this exercise.

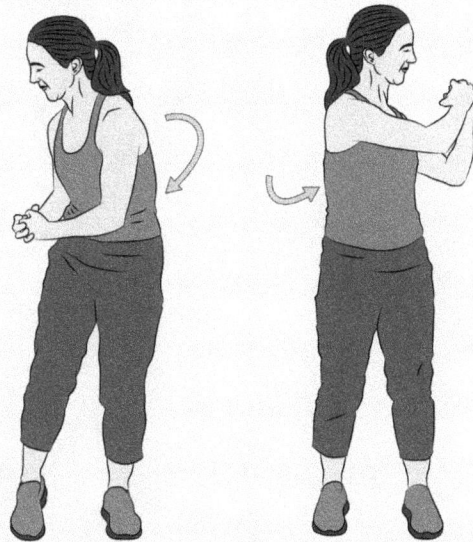

WOOD CHOPS

TIME PER REP: 10 SECONDS | TOTAL TIME: 2 MINUTES

HOW TO:

1. Standing upright with your feet flat on the floor, have a slight bend in your knees.
2. Interlock your fingers as you clasp your hands together. Bring your hands up to, or slightly above, your right shoulder.
3. In one motion, bring your clasped hands down from your right shoulder to the opposite hip. Keep your core tight and engaged as you do this. Repeat five more times.
4. Switch sides by bringing your clasped hands up towards your left shoulder. Move your hands from your left shoulder down to the opposite hip in a single motion. Repeat five more times.

LEVEL UP:

If you have had a shoulder injury or surgery, it may be uncomfortable to have both hands clasped together in this exercise. A variation is to only use one hand. Bring your right hand from your right shoulder down to your opposite hip and vice versa.

TAKE NOTE:

Don't allow your hips to move from side to side. Keep them as stationary as possible.

Chapter 6:
Core Exercises with a Partner

I get by with a little help from my friends.

—The Beatles

Working out with a spouse, partner, helper, or workout buddy is fun and encouraging. It makes the time go quicker and gives us an extra incentive to complete our exercises together. Pick a workout partner that is encouraging, motivated, and consistent. Some of the partner exercises require a bit more strength, but with time and practice, you will be able to do these easily.

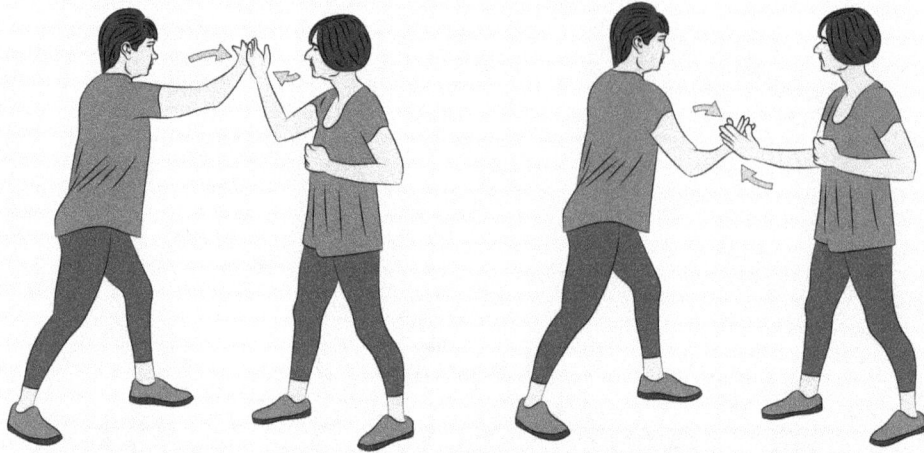

HAND SHADOWING

TIME PER REP: VARIES | TOTAL TIME: 2 MINUTES

HOW TO:

1. Stand face-to-face with your partner. Your feet should be hip-width apart, and knees slightly bent.

2. You and your partner will bend your right arms with elbows at a 90-degree angle. Allow the backs of your hands to touch and firmly press them together.

3. Keeping the backs of you and your partner's hands pressed together in line with the center of your bodies, try to press your partner's hand away as they resist. Move your hand up and down, still trying to press their hand away. Continue for one minute.

4. Switch hands. Now do the exercise with your left hand.

LEVEL UP:

As a variation, you can press your palms together instead of the backs of your hands.

TAKE NOTE:

Tighten your abs each time you move or press your partner's hand.

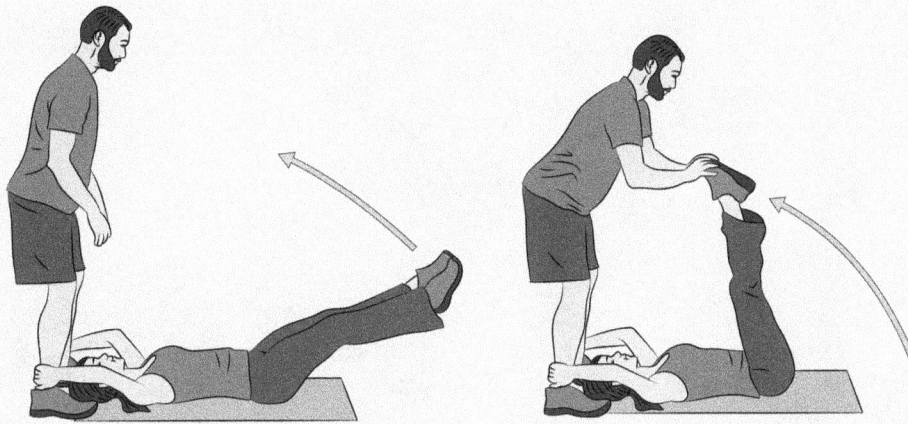

LEG RAISE PUSH DOWN

TIME PER REP: 10 SECONDS | TOTAL TIME: 1 MINUTE

HOW TO:

1. You will lie down on your back on a mat that is on the floor. Your partner will stand with their feet just above your head and facing towards your legs.

2. Raise your arms above your head and, with both hands, grab the outside of their ankles for support.

3. Lift both of your feet off the floor. Bring them up so that they are straight up above your hips. Keep your legs straight or with a slight bend.

4. With their hands, your partner will push both of your feet away. As your feet fall towards the floor, tighten your abdominal muscles to prevent them from reaching the floor and bring them back up above your hips.

5. Your partner will push your feet down again, and you will bring them back up again five more times.

LEVEL UP:

If this is too difficult, start off doing one leg at a time. As you get stronger, you can work your way up to doing both legs together.

TAKE NOTE:

Don't let your lower back arch too much. Try to keep it relaxed but taut.

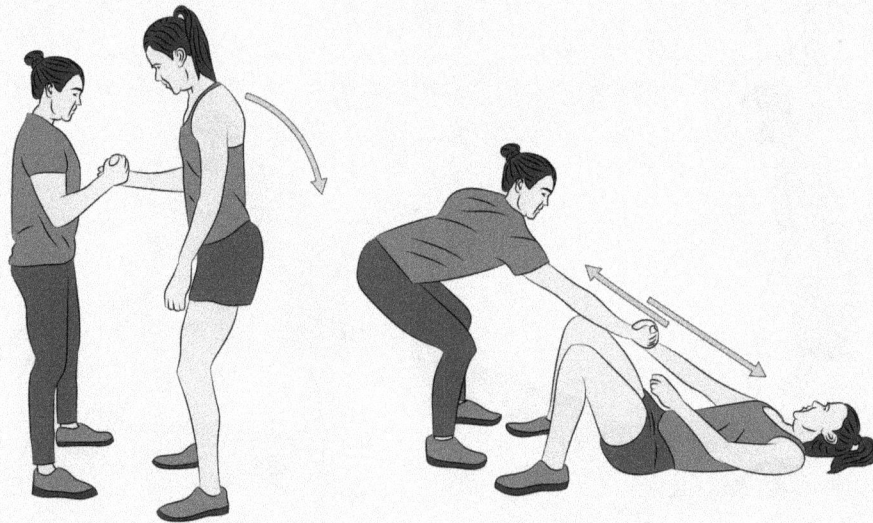

PARTNER GET UP

HOW TO:

1. Lie down on a mat with your knees bent and pointing towards the ceiling. Your partner stands at your feet, facing you.

2. Raise both arms as your partner grabs both of your hands.

3. Using your ab muscles, sit up. Still holding on to your partner's hands, raise yourself up from sitting to standing.

4. Repeat three more times.

LEVEL UP:

To make this more difficult, use only one hand. With your right hand, grab your partner's left hand as you sit up and stand up.

TAKE NOTE:

If you are using only one hand, be sure to do an equal number of moves with the other hand, too.

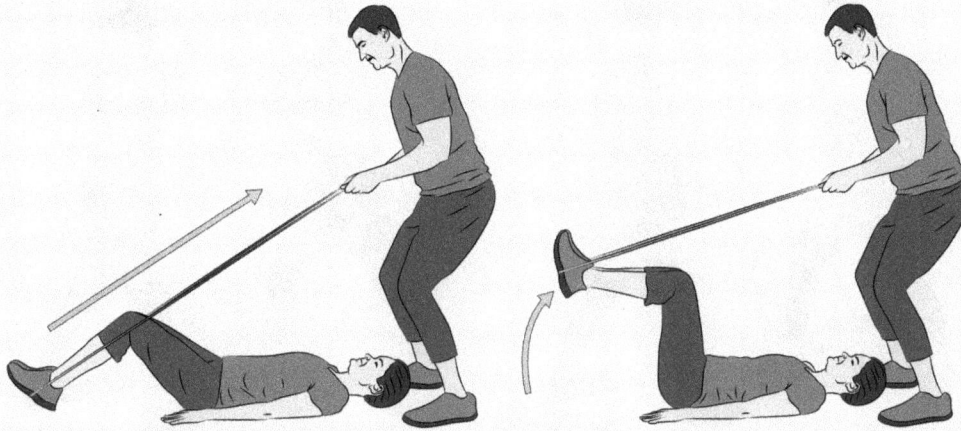

PARTNER HEEL TAP

HOW TO:

1. Lie down on your back on a mat. Your partner will stand with their feet at your head, facing your legs and feet.

2. Loop a resistance band under your feet and bend your knees, so they are pointing towards the ceiling. Your partner will grab the handles of the resistance band.

3. As your partner holds the handles of the band, keep your knees bent and lower your heels to the floor. You will feel your abdominals contract. Once you tap your heels, return your legs to the starting position.

4. Repeat five more times.

LEVEL UP:

As a variation, you can do one leg at a time. Loop the band under one foot as you lower that one to the floor.

TAKE NOTE:

Take care that the band is looped under the middle of your foot (not just looped at the ball of your feet) so that it doesn't slip off and snap towards you or your partner.

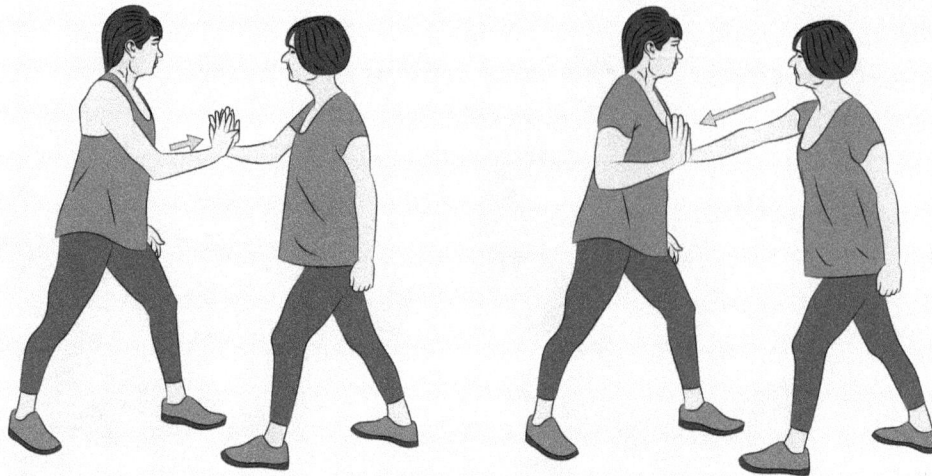

PARTNER PUSH

TIME PER REP: VARIES | TOTAL TIME: 2 MINUTES

HOW TO:

1. Stand tall, facing your partner. Both of you bend your right arms so that your elbows are at a 90-degree angle. With fingers facing up towards the ceiling, press your right palms together.

2. Both of you take a slight step back with your right foot so that your left foot is in front.

3. With right palms pressing towards each other, slowly push your partner's hand back as they gently resist until their hand is almost in line with their chest.

4. Now your partner will slowly push your hand back towards your chest as you resist. Keep going back and forth on this hand for one minute.

5. Switch sides. Do the same exercise with the palms of your left hands pressing against each other. Repeat going back and forth for one minute.

LEVEL UP:

As you get stronger, your partner can resist more strongly against your push.

TAKE NOTE:

Remember to tighten your tummy as you push against each other's palms.

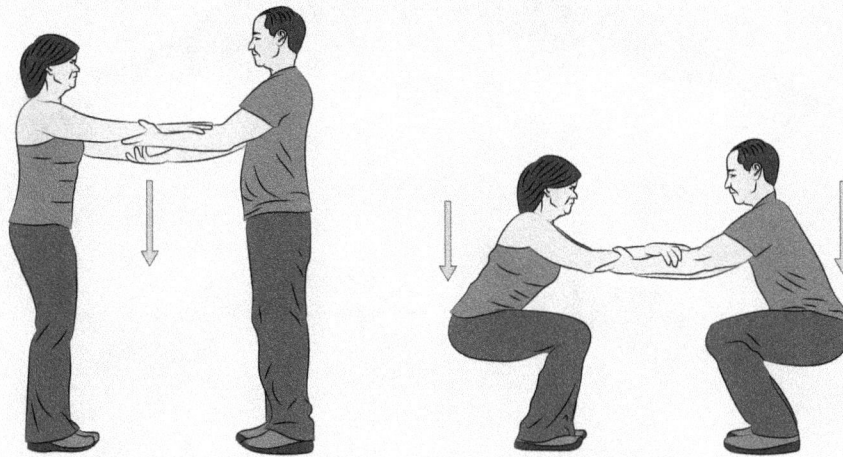

PARTNER SQUAT USING BOTH HANDS

TIME PER REP: 10 SECONDS | TOTAL TIME: 1 MINUTE

HOW TO:

1. Stand upright facing your partner, a few feet apart, with your feet hip-width apart.

2. Grab both hands with your partner. At the same time, both of you lower into a squat. Go as low as is comfortable, then return to standing.

3. Repeat five more times.

LEVEL UP:

To make this harder, only hang on with one hand. Both of you grab each other's right hands and lower into a squat. Be sure to switch sides and do the exercise with your left hands.

TAKE NOTE:

You may find that you can squat a little lower with a partner because of the counterweight balance they provide.

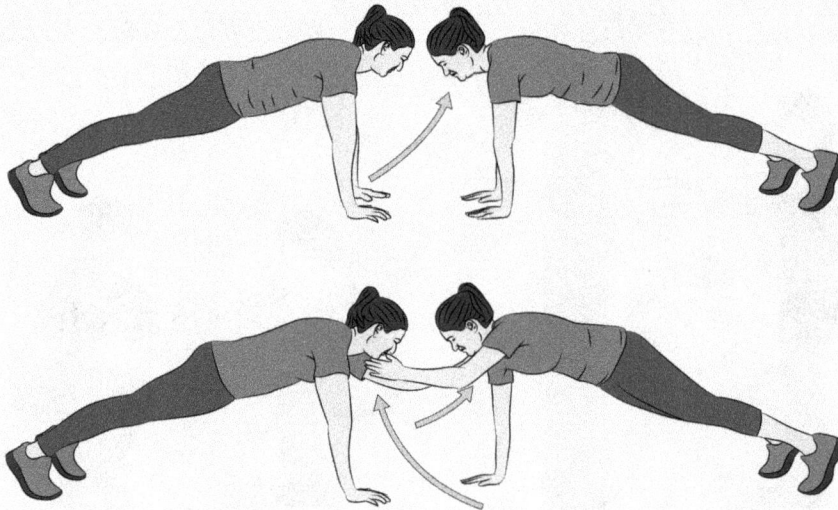

REACH AND TOUCH PLANK

TIME PER REP: 10 SECONDS | TOTAL TIME: 1 MINUTE

HOW TO:

1. Both you and your partner get into a plank position on the mat, facing each other. Your heads should be close and your feet away from each other.

2. You and your partner lift your right hands and touch each other's left shoulder. Alternatively, you can touch each other's right hand. Return to the starting position.

3. Switch sides and lift your left hands and touch each other.

4. Keep switching back and forth until one minute is up.

LEVEL UP:

Depending on your strength, you can do this plank on your knees (a modified plank) or on your toes (regular plank).

TAKE NOTE:

To keep your balance, place your feet slightly wider than normal for extra stability.

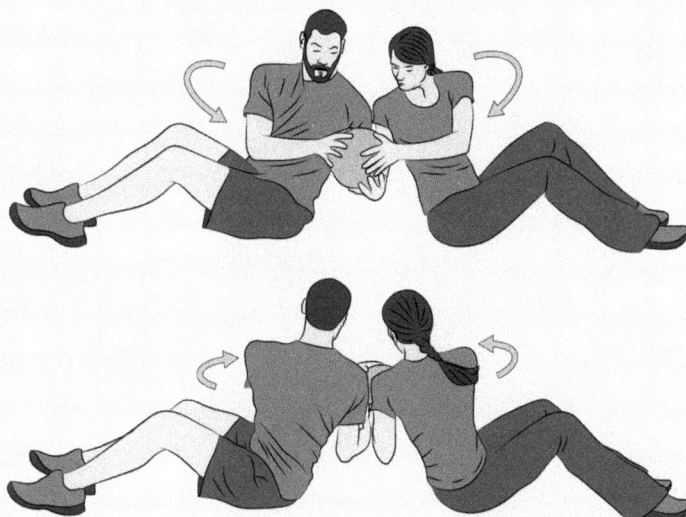

RUSSIAN TWIST AND PASS

TIME PER REP: 5 SECONDS | TOTAL TIME: 2 MINUTES

HOW TO:

1. Sit on a mat back-t0-back with your partner. Both of you bend your legs, so your knees are pointing towards the ceiling.

2. Bend your arms at the elbow with your hands straight out in front of you.

3. Holding a ball, stuffed animal, or small pillow, turn your torso to your right and pass the ball to your partner.

4. Twist your torso to the left to receive the ball back from your partner. Keep turning and passing the ball to your right for one minute.

5. Switch directions. Now pass the ball to your left by twisting your torso to the left. Turn back to the right to receive the ball again. Continue doing this for one minute.

LEVEL UP:

A variation of this can be done while standing. Stand back-to-back and pass the ball in one direction, then switch directions.

TAKE NOTE:

Be sure to tighten your core muscles as you twist from side to side.

Chapter 7:
Warm-Up and Cool Down

I love laugh lines. It means you've had a good life.

—Aerin Lauder

People often forget to warm-up their bodies before doing any exercise. Taking five minutes to get your blood moving and muscles warm will help prevent any strains or injuries. Stretching after exercising is also important as it gives your muscles a chance to relax and stretch while they are warm. This also helps prevent injuries and cramps from happening.

WARM-UP
MOVES

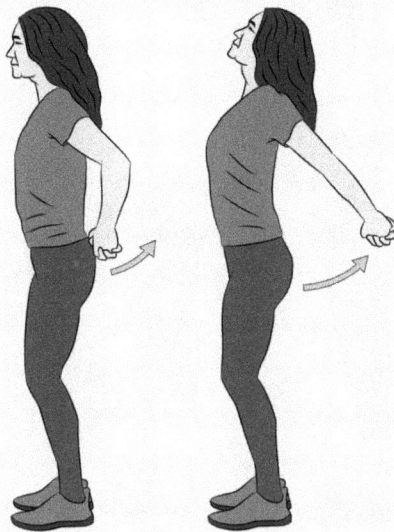

CHEST OPENER

TIME PER REP: 10 SECONDS | TOTAL TIME: 1 MINUTE

HOW TO:

1. Stand up tall with feet hip-width distance apart. Hands are down by your sides.
2. Bring your hands behind you and clasp them together. Straighten both arms as you lift your hands slightly away from your buttocks and push out your chest.
3. Return hands down to the starting position.
4. Repeat five more times.

TAKE NOTE:

If you cannot clasp your hands behind you, it is okay. You can bring both hands behind you as you lift your arms as high as you can while pushing out your chest.

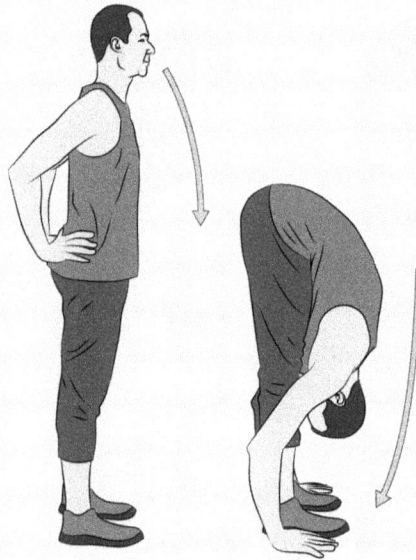

FORWARD FOLD

TIME PER REP: 15 SECONDS | TOTAL TIME: 1 MINUTE

HOW TO:

1. Stand with your feet hip-width distance apart and hands down by your sides.
2. As you inhale, raise both arms and bring your hands above your head.
3. On the exhale, bend forward at the waist and bring your hands down towards the floor. Let your head hang and be heavy as your back muscles stretch out.
4. Slowly roll back up to starting position. Repeat three more times.

TAKE NOTE:

Your legs don't have to be perfectly straight as you do this. It is okay if they are slightly bent.

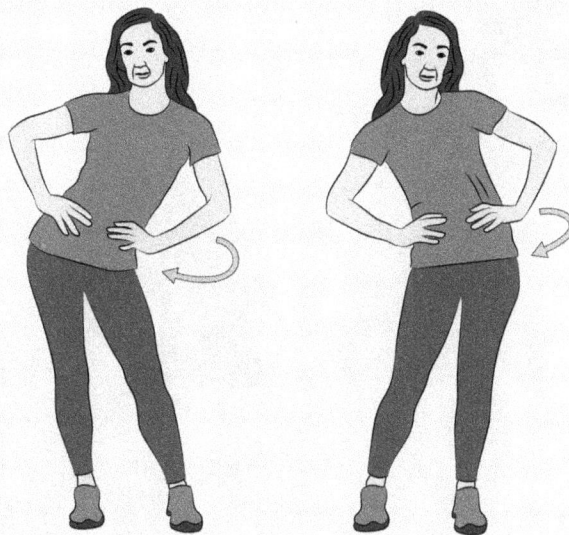

HIP CIRCLES

HOW TO:

1. Stand with your feet hip-width distance apart, and knees slightly bent.
2. Place your hands on your hips.
3. Move your hips forward, right, back, and left. Repeat moving them in a clockwise motion for 30 seconds.
4. Switch directions and now move your hips counter-clockwise for another 30 seconds.

TAKE NOTE:

As you get warmed up, your hips will begin to move in a larger circle.

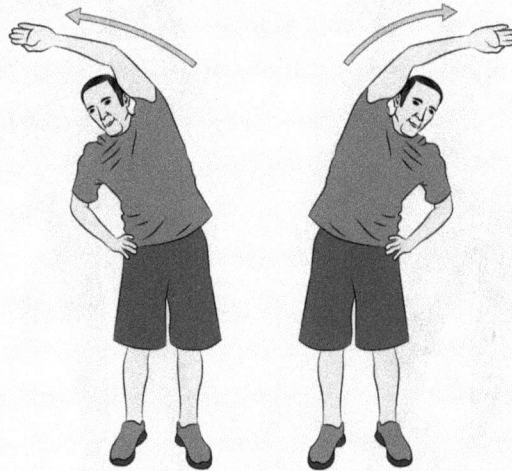

SIDE REACH

TIME PER REP: 5 SECONDS | TOTAL TIME: 1 MINUTE

HOW TO:

1. Stand erect with your feet hip-width distant apart. Hands are down by your sides.

2. Raise your right arm and bring your right hand over your head as you bend your torso to the left. Bring the arm down and return to the starting position.

3. Switch sides and raise your left arm up as you bend to the right. Return to the starting position.

4. Alternate bending right and then left for one minute.

TAKE NOTE:

Keep your chest facing straight in front of you as you bend from side to side.

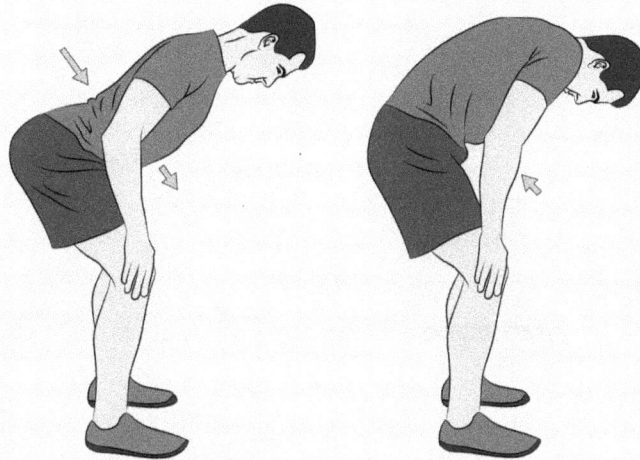

STANDING CAT COW

TIME PER REP: 10 SECONDS | TOTAL TIME: 1 MINUTE

HOW TO:

1. Stand with your feet slightly wider than hip-width apart and knees bent.
2. Bend forward and place your hands on the tops of your knees.
3. Take a breath, inhaling as you drop your chin towards your chest and round your upper back (this is the cat position).
4. Exhale as you lift your chin to look up and arch your back, allowing your belly to relax towards your thighs (cow position).
5. Repeat the moves, alternating between cat and cow, for one minute.

TAKE NOTE:

Keep your shoulders relaxed throughout this warm-up exercise, and don't hunch up.

COOL DOWN
STRETCHES

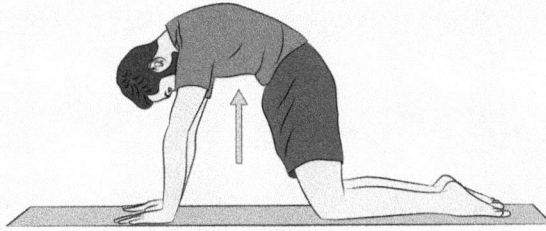

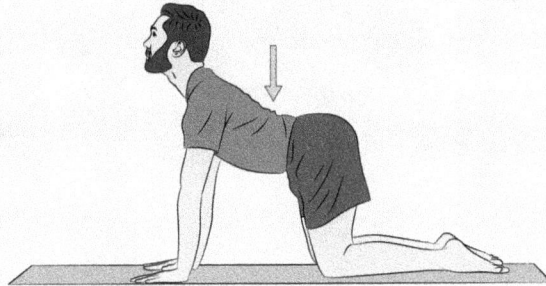

CAT COW

HOW TO:

1. Get on your hands and knees on a mat on the floor. Hands are directly under your shoulders and knees directly under your hips.
2. Take a breath, inhaling as you drop your chin towards your chest and round your upper back (cat position).
3. Exhale as you lift your chin to look up and arch your back, allowing your belly to relax towards the floor (cow position).
4. Repeat the moves, alternating between cat and cow, for one minute.

TAKE NOTE:

Pay attention to any tightness in your upper and lower back. Adjust your stretch to accommodate your mobility in these areas.

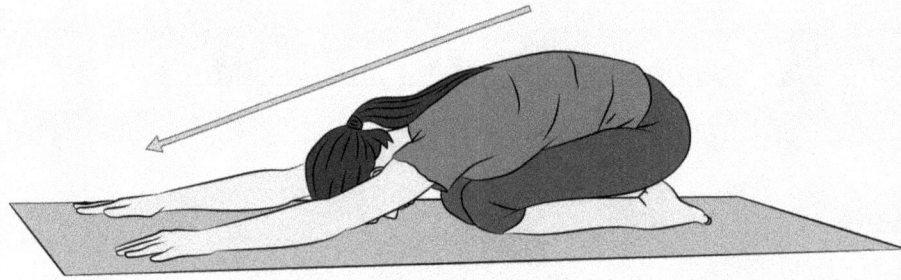

CHILD'S POSE

HOW TO:

1. Get on your hands and knees on a mat on the floor. Keeping your big toes together, widen your knees apart as far as comfortable.

2. Lower your hips to your feet while lowering your upper body and forehead down to the mat. Arms are out in front of you, reaching above your head, and hands are on the floor. Breathe in and out as you relax in this position for 10 seconds. Return to the starting position.

3. Repeat two more times.

TAKE NOTE:

If you have shoulder issues, it may be more comfortable for you to have your arms alongside your torso. Arms are resting on the floor with your palms facing up to the ceiling.

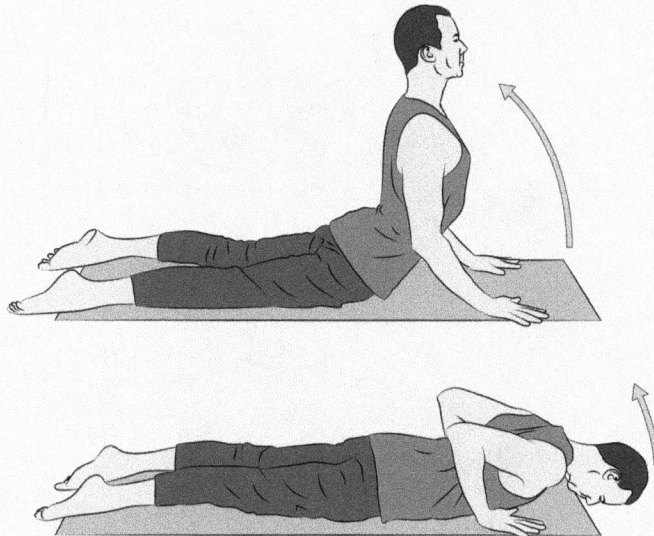

COBRA

HOW TO:

1. Lie down on a mat, face down, with your stomach on the mat. Legs are straight behind you, and the soles of the feet are facing up towards the ceiling.

2. Place your hands under your shoulders, palms down on the floor.

3. Press into your hands as you straighten your arms while raising your head and upper torso off the floor. Keep your hips pressed to the mat. Gently lower down to the starting position.

4. Repeat three more times.

TAKE NOTE:

It might be more comfortable for you to simply prop yourself up with your forearms on the floor rather than straightening your arms.

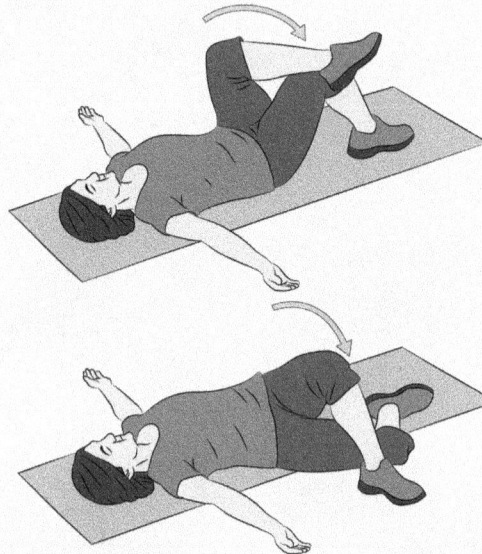

LEG CROSSOVER

HOW TO:

1. Lie down with your back on the mat. Bend your knees, so they are pointing towards the ceiling. Bring your arms out into a T-position with your palms facing up.

2. Bring your right foot up and place it on top of your left knee. If needed, you can use your right hand to gently push your right knee away from you. Hold this position for five seconds.

3. Allow your left leg to slowly fall over to the left side and sole of your right foot to touch the floor, if possible. You might not be able to cross over all the way, and that's okay. Return to the starting position.

4. Switch legs. Place your left foot on your right knee. Let your right leg fall to the right, and your left sole to touch the floor. Return to starting positions and repeat once on each side.

TAKE NOTE:

Keep your chest facing up towards the ceiling at all times and the back of both shoulders firmly planted on the floor.

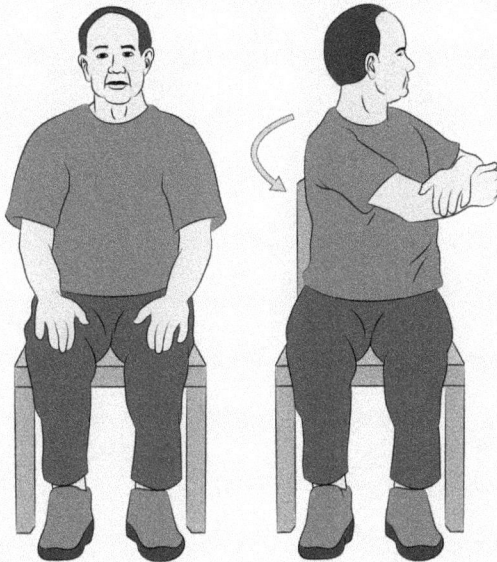

SEATED ROTATION

TIME PER REP: 15 SECONDS | TOTAL TIME: 1 MINUTE

HOW TO:

1. From a seated position, either in a chair or on the floor, sit up tall.

2. Cross your arms in front of you, keeping your shoulders relaxed.

3. Keeping your hips facing forward, turn your arms and upper torso to the right and look over your right shoulder. Hold this position for five seconds, then return to the starting position.

4. Now, turn your arms and torso to the left as you look over your left shoulder. Hold for five seconds, then return to the starting position.

5. Repeat the exercise once more on each side.

TAKE NOTE:

If you have had a neck injury or surgery, keep your head in line with your upper torso and don't look over your shoulder.

Chapter 8:
Walking Core Exercises

Walking is man's best medicine.

—Hippocrates

Walking is a great way to get in some cardiovascular exercise, breathe in fresh air, and loosen muscles. It is a chance to get outdoors, enjoy the sunshine, and take in new views. Walking is also an opportunity to spend social time with others as you exercise together and build friendships. There are several core exercises that can be done while walking. While no equipment is needed, you can choose to add lightweight hand weights if you choose to.

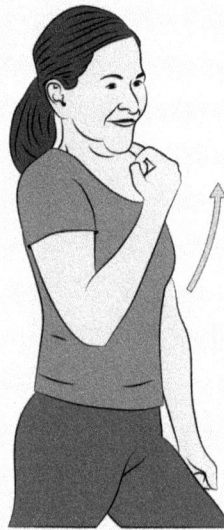

ARM CURLS

HOW TO:

1. Bend your arms at the elbows so that they form a 90-degree angle.
2. Slowly lower both hands down, then raise them up towards your shoulders. This is the same motion as doing a bicep curl.
3. Repeat the arm curls for one minute.

LEVEL UP:

To make this more difficult, you can add one or two-pound weights in each hand.

TAKE NOTE:

Make this a slow and controlled movement. Don't pump your arms up and down.

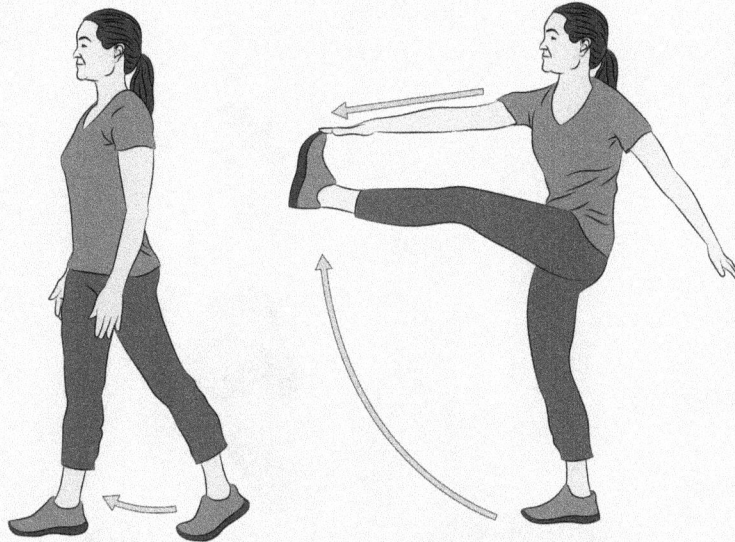

LEG LIFT TOE TOUCHES

TIME PER REP: VARIES | TOTAL TIME: 1 MINUTE

HOW TO:

1. Keeping it straight, lift your right leg as high as you can. At the same time, reach with your left hand towards your raised right foot as you twist your torso to the right. This requires some balance. Return to the starting position.

2. Switch legs. Lift your left leg and reach towards it with your opposite hand.

3. Continue to walk forward, lifting alternate legs, for one minute.

LEVEL UP:

A variation of this is to lift just your knee instead of your entire leg.

TAKE NOTE:

Be sure you are walking on a level floor free from rocks and other things you could stumble over while doing this exercise.

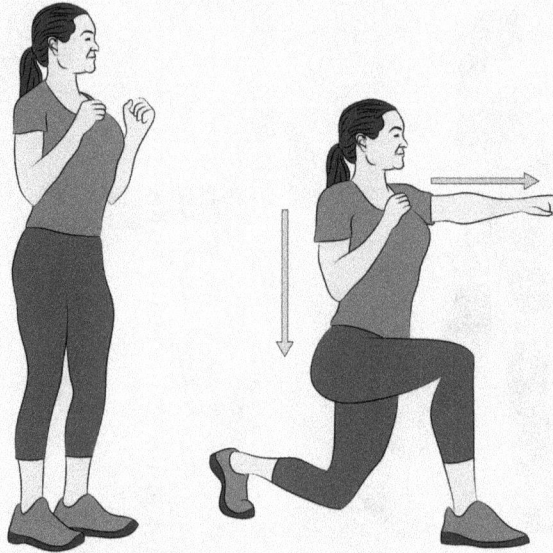

PUNCH FORWARD

TIME PER REP: VARIES | TOTAL TIME: 1 MINUTE

HOW TO:

1. Make a fist with both hands. Bring both hands up to the sides of your chest.
2. Punch your right fist out in front of you, slightly to the left of your torso and twisting your body slightly to the left. Bring your arm back.
3. Now, punch your left fist to the right of your torso and twist slightly to the right.
4. Repeat punching forward, alternating arms, for one minute.

LEVEL UP:

You can make this more challenging by adding one or two-pound weights in each hand.

TAKE NOTE:

Be sure to tighten your abs and exhale as you punch each time.

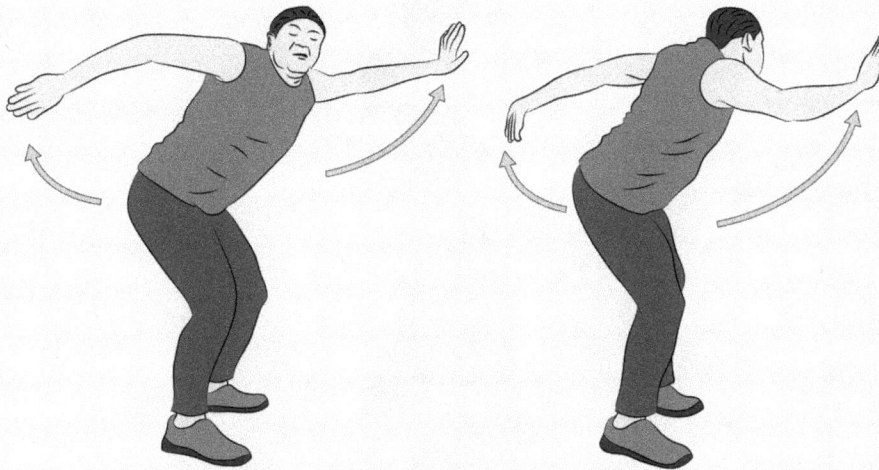

SWING YOUR ARMS

TIME PER REP: VARIES | TOTAL TIME: 1 MINUTE

HOW TO:

1. Bend your arms at the elbow, so they are at 90-degree angles.
2. As your right foot steps forward, swing your bent left arm forward.
3. When your left foot steps forward, swing your right arm forward.
4. Keep walking forward, swinging the opposite arm forward to help propel you along.

LEVEL UP:

Adding one or two-pound weights in each hand will make this more difficult.

TAKE NOTE:

Ensure that whatever foot is forward, the opposite arm is forward. Having the same foot and arm forward at the same time will result in an awkward gait.

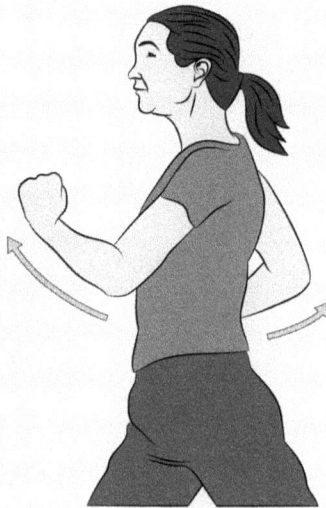

TIGHTEN YOUR TUMMY

TIME PER REP: VARIES | TOTAL TIME: 1 MINUTE INTERVALS

HOW TO:

1.   As you walk, draw in your abdominal muscles and lift your chest.
2.   Keep these muscles engaged for one minute or as long as you can.
3.   Repeat the exercise a few times during your walk.

LEVEL UP:

You can place your hand on your belly as a reminder to keep your core engaged as you walk.

TAKE NOTE:

Keep your shoulders relaxed and maintain good posture as you tighten your core muscles.

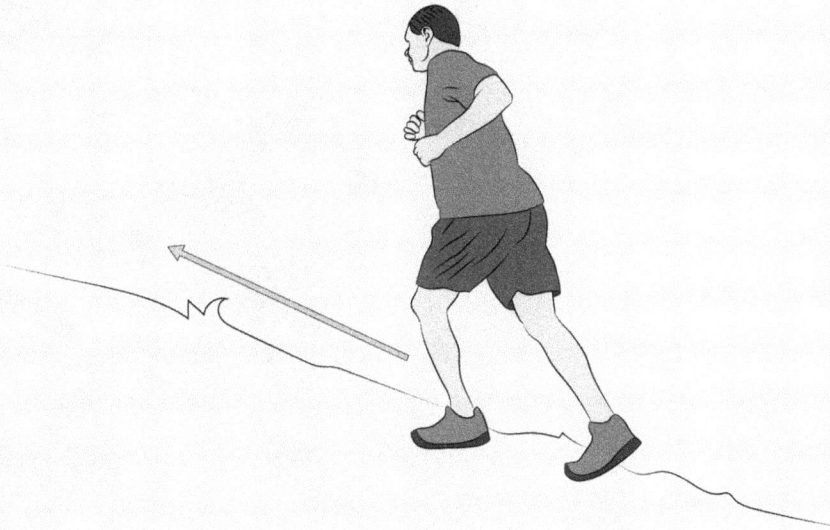

WALK UPHILL

TIME PER REP: VARIES | TOTAL TIME: VARIES

HOW TO:

1. Find a walking path that includes an incline or uphill section.
2. As you walk up the incline, swing your arms to help propel you up the hill. Engage your buttock muscles and tighten your abdominals as you trek the incline.

LEVEL UP:

Incorporating an incline into your walks several times a week will make your walks more challenging.

TAKE NOTE:

Don't lean your chest too far forward as you walk uphill. Maintain good posture and a relaxed neck and upper back.

Chapter 9:
Weekly Schedules

The secret of your future is hidden in your daily routine.

—Mike Murdock

It is time to put all you have learned into an action plan! In this chapter, you will find weekly schedules that incorporate the core exercises into easy-to-follow plans.

There are three weeks of routines, six days per week. This leaves room for rest days and for the unexpected day off. Many people believe that twenty-one days of doing something builds a new habit. In reality, it takes longer than that, but three weeks is a good kick-start towards your goal of a stronger core and improved stability as you age.

- Five days start with a warm-up exercise, include three core exercises, and end with a cool down exercise.

- There is a daily focus of either mat, seated, or standing moves.

- One day is devoted to walking and the core exercises that accompany it.

- If you have a partner available, you can do the partner exercise as well.

WEEK 1 SCHEDULE

DAY 1

Warm-up: Side Reach

Mat Core Exercises: Dead Bug, Mountain Climber, Superman

Partner Exercise: Partner Reach and Touch Plank

Cool down: Child's Pose

DAY 2

Warm-up: Chest Opener

Seated Core Exercises: Seated Side Bend, Forward Roll Up, Seated Leg Lift

Partner Exercise: Partner Russian Twist and Pass

Cool down: Cobra

DAY 3

Warm-up: Forward Fold

Standing Core Exercises: Standing Bird Dog, Figure 8 Row, Squat

Partner Exercise: Partner Squat with Both Hands

Cool down: Cat Cow

DAY 4

Warm-up: Hip Circles

Mat Core Exercises: Modified Curl Up, Segment Rotation, Plank

Partner Exercise: Partner Leg Raise Push Down

Cool down: Seated Rotation

DAY 5

Warm-up: Standing Cat Cow

Seated Core Exercises: Seated Twist, Half Roll Back, Single Knee Tuck

Partner Exercise: Partner Heel Tap

Cool down: Leg Crossover Stretch

DAY 6 - WALK

Warm-up: Side Reach

Walking Exercises: Swing Your Arms, Walk Uphill

Cool down: Child's Pose

WEEK 2 SCHEDULE

DAY 1

Warm-up: Chest Opener

Standing Core Exercises: Standing Side Bend, Core Rotation, Knee Rotation

Partner Exercise: Partner Push

Cool down: Cobra

DAY 2

Warm-up: Forward Fold

Mat Core Exercises: Bridge, Side Plank, Single Leg Abdominal Press

Partner Exercise: Partner Get Ups

Cool down: Cat Cow

DAY 3

Warm-up: Hip Circles

Seated Core Exercises: Seated Dead Bug, Leg Taps, Seated Russian Twist

Partner Exercise: Partner Hand Shadows

Cool down: Leg Crossover Stretch

DAY 4

Warm-up: Standing Cat Cow

Standing Core Exercises: Standing Twist, Standing Bicycle Crunch, Wide Side Crunch

Partner Exercise: Partner Squat with Both Hands

Cool down: Seated Rotation

DAY 5

Warm-up: Side Reach

Mat Core Exercises: Bird Dog, Side Plank with Rotation, Supine Toe Tap

Partner Exercise: Partner Reach and Touch Plank

Cool down: Child's Pose

DAY 6 - WALK

Warm-up: Chest Opener

Walking Exercises: Punch Forward, Tighten Your Tummy

Cool down: Cobra

WEEK 3 SCHEDULE

DAY 1

Warm-up: Forward Fold

Seated Core Exercises: Band Extension, Resisted Knee Lift, Seated Jumping Jack

Partner Exercise: Partner Heel Tap

Cool down: Leg Crossover Stretch

DAY 2

Warm-up: Hip Circles

Standing Core Exercises: Standing Crunch, Knee Tuck Extension, Woodchops

Partner Exercise: Partner Hand Shadow

Cool down: Seated Rotation

DAY 3

Warm-up: Standing Cat Cow

Mat Core Exercises: Dead Bug, Mountain Climber, Superman

Partner Exercise: Partner Russian Twist and Pass

Cool down: Cat Cow

DAY 4

Warm-up: Side Reach

Seated Core Exercises: Seated Side Bend, Forward Roll-Up, Seated Leg Lift

Partner Exercise: Partner Leg Raise Push Down

Cool down: Child's Pose

DAY 5

Warm-up: Chest Opener

Standing Core Exercises: Standing Bird Dog, Figure 8 Row, Squat

Partner Exercise: Partner Get Up

Cool down: Cobra

DAY 6 - WALK

Warm-up: Forward Fold

Walking Exercises: Arm Curls, Leg Lift Toe Touches

Cool down: Leg Crossover Stretch

CONCLUSION

You made it! Congratulations on taking charge of your health and well-being by choosing to learn how to age well. As we have traveled this journey together, we have discovered a lot about our bodies and how they function. So, many factors contribute to how our bodies respond to the number of years we live on this earth. Some elements we cannot control, but those that we can include diet, exercise, and the choices we make.

One of the pillars of aging well is having a core of strength and flexibility. Because our core muscles are responsible for our ability to accomplish everyday tasks, engage in physical activities, and even play with our grandchildren. They play an essential role in our overall vitality. Early on in the book, we looked at the disadvantages of having a weak core versus the advantages of maintaining a strong one. Then, we assessed the state of our core strengths and weaknesses with a simple quiz.

The following chapters outlined a variety of core exercises that can immediately be put into practice. The core exercises we learned comprised of:

- Mat core exercises. These twelve exercises are done close to the floor on all fours or lying down and help us increase our ability to get up and down more easily.

- Seated core exercises. Able to be done by those who have trouble standing or getting on the floor, these twelve exercises helped us build our core strength from a seated position.

- Standing core exercises. Balance and stability are significant components in core strength and working through the twelve standing exercises helped train our muscles for everyday activities.

- Partner core exercises. These eight exercises added a little fun and encouragement as we worked on our core with a workout partner.

- Warm-up and cool down. Often overlooked, these warm-ups and cool down stretches help our muscles transition from inactivity to activity and back.

- Walking core exercises. Doing double duty, these exercises work the core muscles and can be done while getting in a walk.

97

Finally, we looked at incorporating all that we have learned into a weekly workout schedule. Depending on your preferences and goals, you can work through each exercise at your own pace, doing one a day, until you work through all fifty exercises. For those looking for a ready-made plan, the daily routines listed provide an easy way to complete the exercises in this book without having to come up with your plan.

My hope and desire is that you will benefit from the information and encouragement in this book. If you found this book helpful, please consider leaving a review and letting me know your thoughts! I look forward to hearing how implementing these exercises into your daily plan of exercise and wellness helps you build strength and stability in your core.

Scan the QR Code To Leave a Review:

I hope you enjoy good health and happiness on the long road ahead of you, and I wish you all the best. Thank you for allowing me to s share my knowledge with you.

Baz Thompson

REFERENCES

5 Core Exercises for Seniors: Build Strength From Your Center. (n.d.). Retrieved February 19, 2022, from Snug Safety website: http://www.snugsafe.com/all-posts/core-exercises-for-seniors

6 Core Stretches That Will Make Your Abs Feel Amazing. (n.d.). Retrieved February 19, 2022, from LIVESTRONG.COM website: http://www.livestrong.com/article/355186-core-muscle-stretches

Arana, J. (2020, June 25). How to Tone Abs While Walking. Retrieved February 19, 2022, from wikiHow website: http://www.wikihow.com/Tone-Abs-While-Walking

Back Exercises: Neck and Torso Rotation. (n.d.). Retrieved February 19, 2022, from demo.staywellhealthlibrary.com website: https://demo.staywellhealthlibrary.com/Content/healthsheets-v1/neck-exercises-necktorso-rotation/

Barroa_Artworks. (2022). Retrieved February 15, 2022, from Pixabay.com website: https://cdn.pixabay.com/photo/2018/01/31/07/53/muscle-3120521_960_720.png

Bedosky, L. (2021, March 13). The Best Core Exercises for Seniors. Retrieved from Get Healthy U | Chris Freytag website: https://gethealthyu.com/best-core-exercises-for-seniors/

Bubnis, D. (2016, February 11). 29 Full-Body Partner Exercises. Retrieved February 19, 2022, from Greatist website: https://greatist.com/fitness/35-kick-ass-partner-exercises

Bubnis, D. (2020, April 11). When's the Best Time to Exercise? Retrieved February 13, 2022, from Greatist website: https://greatist.com/fitness/whats-best-time-work-out

Capritto, A. (2020, November 24). 4 important benefits of a strong core. Retrieved February 13, 2022, from CNET website: https://www.cnet.com/health/fitness/why-you-really-need-a-strong-core-for-fitness-and-life/

Davis, N. (2020, October 23). Try This: 24 Standing Ab Exercises to Strengthen and Define Your Core. Retrieved February 19, 2022, from Healthline website: https://www.healthline.com/health/fitness-exercise/standing-ab-exercises#stretch.

Dilthey, M. R. (2020, January 23). Is It Better to Do Your Ab Workout in the Morning or at Night? Retrieved from LIVESTRONG.COM website: https://www.livestrong.com/article/301734-the-best-time-to-work-out-abs/

Exercise Library:Cobra. (n.d.). Retrieved from www.acefitness.org website: https://www.acefitness.org/education-and-resources/lifestyle/exercise-library/16/cobra/

Exercise Library:Leg Crossover Stretch. (n.d.). Retrieved February 10, 2022, from www.acefitness.org website: https://www.acefitness.org/education-and-resources/lifestyle/exercise-library/231/leg-crossover-stretch/

Ferraro, K. (2021, September 11). The 10 Benefits of a Strong Core, According to Trainers. Retrieved from Byrdie website: https://www.byrdie.com/benefits-of-a-strong-core-5189502

Fetters, A. (2017, September 25). The 10-Minute Seated Core Workout. Retrieved February 19, 2022, from SilverSneakers website: http://www.silversneakers.com/blog/10-minute-chair-core-workout

Fetters, A. (2019, March 12). 6 Core Exercises to Ease Lower Back Pain. Retrieved February 19, 2022, from SilverSneakers website: http://www.silversneakers.com/blog/core-exercises-ease-back-pain

Harvard Health, P. (2012, January 12). The real-world benefits of strengthening your core. Retrieved from Harvard Health website: https://www.health.harvard.edu/healthbeat/the-real-world-benefits-of-strengthening-your-core

Kissam, B. (2018, September 17). 0-6 Pack Abs Phase 1 - Miracle Muscles | Warrior Made. Retrieved February 19, 2022, from results.warriormade.com website: https://results.warriormade.com/0-6pack-abs/phase1-miracle-muscles/

Lefkowith, C. (2015, July 22). 20 Partner Exercises | Redefining Strength. Retrieved from Redefining Strength website: https://redefiningstrength.com/try-these-20-partner-exercises-for-a-fun-full-body-workout/

Malacoff, J. (2018, April 24). 6 Signs You Need to Strengthen Your Core | Fitness | MyFitnessPal. Retrieved from MyFitnessPal Blog website: https://blog.myfitnesspal.com/6-signs-you-need-to-strengthen-your-core/

Maurice. (2021, February 1). Core Exercises for Seniors: Complete Guide to Ab Exercises for Seniors -. Retrieved from Seniors Mobility website: https://seniorsmobility.org/exercises/core-exercises-for-seniors/

McCormick, R., & Vasilaki, A. (2018). Age-related changes in skeletal muscle: changes to life-style as a therapy. Biogerontology, 19(6), 519–536. https://doi.org/10.1007/s10522-018-9775-3

Miller, B. (2016, January 29). 6 Ways To Tone Your Abs While You Walk. Retrieved from Prevention website: https://www.prevention.com/fitness/a20496857/tone-your-abs-while-walking/

Moreland, B., Kakara, R., & Henry, A. (2020). Trends in Nonfatal Falls and Fall-Related Injuries Among Adults Aged ≤65 Years — United States, 2012–2018. MMWR. Morbidity and Mortality Weekly Report, 69(27), 875–881. https://doi.org/10.15585/mmwr.mm6927a5

Nunez, K. (2021, September 27). Best Core Exercises: Top Moves, from Beginner to Advanced. Retrieved February 19, 2022, from Healthline website: https://www.healthline.com/health/best-core-exercises#Bicycle-crunch.

Partner Workout with Kelli & Daniel - Fitness Blender's 100th Free Full Length Workout Video. (2012, July 9). Retrieved February 19, 2022, from www.youtube.com website: http://www.youtube.com/watch?v=tD-4Vm0AY28

Pizer, A. (2020, March 27). The Child's Pose for Resting in Yoga. Retrieved from Verywell Fit website: https://www.verywellfit.com/childs-pose-balasana-3567066

Pizer, A. (2021, December 8). How to Do Cat-Cow Stretch (Chakravakasana) in Yoga. Retrieved from Verywell Fit website: https://www.verywellfit.com/cat-cow-stretch-chakravakasana-3567178

Search Results. (n.d.). Retrieved February 12, 2022, from BrainyQuote website: https://www.brainyquote.com/search_results?x=0&y=0&q=aging+strong

Slide show: Exercises to improve your core strength. (2020, August 11). Retrieved from Mayo Clinic website: https://www.mayoclinic.org/healthy-lifestyle/fitness/multimedia/core-strength/sls-20076575?s=8

The best core exercises for older adults. (2021, April 1). Retrieved from Harvard Health website: https://www.health.harvard.edu/staying-healthy/the-best-core-exercises-for-older-adults

Townsend, H. (2020, June 16). 7 Standing Core Exercises for Seniors. Retrieved February 19, 2022, from SilverSneakers website: https://www.silversneakers.com/blog/7-standing-exercises-for-core-strength

www.ingramcontent.com/pod-product-compliance
Lightning Source LLC
Chambersburg PA
CBHW052116020426
42335CB00021B/2792